POCKET GUIDE TO DIAGNOSTIC CARDIAC CATHETERIZATION

Andro G. Kacharava, MD, PhD

Stephen D. Clements Jr., MD

A. Maziar Zafari, MD, PhD

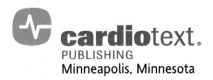

PUBLISHING
Minneapolis, Minnesota

© 2016 Andro G. Kacharava, Stephen D. Clements Jr., A. Maziar Zafari

Cardiotext Publishing, LLC
3405 W. 44th Street
Minneapolis, Minnesota 55410
USA

www.cardiotextpublishing.com

Any updates to this book may be found at: www.cardiotextpublishing.com/
pocket-guide-to-diagnostic-cardiac-catheterization

Comments, inquiries, and requests for bulk sales can be directed to the publisher
at: info@cardiotextpublishing.com.

Library of Congress Control Number: 2015950378

ISBN: 978-1-935395-35-5

Printed in the United States of America

Dedicated to
all Emory Cardiology Fellows, past and present

Table of Contents

About the Authors

Andro G. Kacharava, MD, PhD
Assistant Professor of Medicine, Division of Cardiology,
Department of Medicine, Emory University School of Medicine;
Staff Cardiologist, Atlanta Veterans Affairs Medical Center,
Atlanta, Georgia

Stephen D. Clements Jr., MD
Professor of Medicine, R. Harold Harrison Endowed Chair in
Cardiology, Division of Cardiology, Department of Medicine,
Emory University School of Medicine, Atlanta, Georgia

A. Maziar Zafari, MD, PhD, FACC, FAHA
Professor of Medicine, Division of Cardiology, Department
of Medicine, Emory University School of Medicine; Chief of
Cardiology, Atlanta Veterans Affairs Medical Center, Atlanta,
Georgia

Foreword

Diagnostic cardiac catheterization and angiography have been underappreciated for 30 years—and it is our fault!

The expansion of interventional cardiology has resulted in the pure diagnostic catheterizer becoming an endangered species. With the advances in noninvasive imaging, many questions can be answered without inserting catheters, but many others cannot; diagnostic catheterization is not only needed but in many conditions, it is often the most definitive and cost-effective investigation we have.

I defended this position in developing the recent Core Cardiovascular Training Statement (COCATS) documents for training in cardiology, and indeed, it remains a cornerstone for trainees, be they headed for invasive disciplines or not. Today, fellows diving into their cath lab rotations have limited time to absorb all the nuances of how to effectively and safely perform and interpret catheterization procedures. Their instructors are most often interventional cardiologists who may view the diagnostic procedure as only a prologue to what they are most interested in—the intervention.

The *Pocket Guide to Diagnostic Cardiac Catheterization* (which is a modest title for so rich a resource) has the potential to bring fellows up to speed on the first day in the lab and will make the mentoring during the rotation much easier to comprehend. Of the authors, one (SC), who has been my colleague for 40 years, has been dedicated to the performance of diagnostic catheterization predominantly in the outpatient setting. Despite the fact that all interventional cardiologists perform diagnostic procedures, the perspective of the diagnostic-only catheterizer is particularly valuable for trainees.

This book takes the reader from the rudimentary pioneering efforts to the most modern methods. The highly practical approach to addressing the various techniques in catheterization and coronary arteriography is especially valuable and is developed from decades of experience. The reader will find the figures not only beautiful but highly illustrative in their simplicity.

One of our fellows once gave me a bumper sticker emblazoned, "Real men use multipurpose catheters." Some may find the chapter on the multipurpose technique unusual, as most teach the use of preformed catheter approaches to coronary arteriography. I am pleased that this technique, which I introduced at Emory in 1972 and which has been taught to hundreds of trainees over the years, is still alive and breathing. Although it is indeed more difficult, mastering the skills of manipulation of catheters in the aortic root can overcome some of the limitations of fixed preformed devices.

The authors are dedicated to the safe and effective utilization of catheterization for diagnostic purposes, and they have produced a volume that should be a staple for fellows entering a cath lab rotation and a constant source for maintaining their competence in performing and/or interpreting catheterization throughout their careers.

–Spencer B. King III, MD, MACC

Preface

The idea of writing this *Pocket Guide to Diagnostic Cardiac Catheterization* came during the early fellowship years when, despite all good efforts by the cardiology teaching faculty to provide fellows with a formidable teaching milieu, the quality of the teaching process in the busy cardiac catheterization laboratories needed improvement. As first-year fellows, we were overcoming these shortcomings by discussing the patients presented to the laboratory with one another, asking senior fellows for guidance, and of course, reading textbooks about cardiac catheterization and invasive cardiology. Most major textbooks were available to us, but time for junior fellows was a rare commodity; we were trying to find an efficient way to do the job in the cardiac catheterization laboratory and study the essential material quickly. One challenge was the size of the major cardiac catheterization textbooks. Practical pearls of wisdom about the technical aspects of cardiac catheterization and other invasive cardiology procedures for general cardiology fellows were scattered between the lines in many textbooks within the discipline of clinical cardiology and its subspecialties. From a practical standpoint, a *Pocket Guide* enabling fellows to find and review the practical knowledge hidden in the larger textbooks was sorely needed.

This *Pocket Guide*, with step-by-step instructions and easy-to-follow illustrations, was written in response to this need to guide and explain the practical aspects of the various procedures in invasive cardiology and cardiac catheterization. We intend with this *Pocket Guide* to provide trainees with practical knowledge to make their daily and complex duties in the cardiac catheterization laboratory more educational. The rotation in the cardiac catheterization laboratory is, at times, intimidating, and we intend to make this a highly educational and rewarding experience from the beginning of the rotation.

To create this *Pocket Guide*, we have collected most of the practical pearls about cardiac catheterization and various procedures from invasive cardiology textbooks, medical journals, and through our personal experiences in different cardiac catheterization laboratories, where we have worked shoulder-to-shoulder with trainees, teachers, and colleagues. A unique feature of our *Pocket Guide* is a special chapter with video clips that has been created to highlight the role and technical versatility of the multipurpose catheter in cardiac catheterization—a technique developed, taught, and learned over many generations in the cardiac catheterization laboratories at Emory University.

The primary goal of this *Pocket Guide* is to provide general cardiology fellows worldwide who are entering the cardiac catheterization laboratory a practical guide addressing key aspects of cardiac catheterization as learned and taught by the authors. This *Pocket Guide* may be useful as a quick reference for general cardiologists, who are starting their independent practice in academic or private settings as well as cardiac catheterization laboratory technicians and nurses who may want to acquire practical knowledge as it relates to their daily practice. This *Pocket Guide* is not designed to replace textbooks on the subject matter, however; cardiology fellows and other professionals working in the cardiac catheterization laboratory are strongly encouraged to study the comprehensive knowledge and detailed information needed to practice high-quality and safe patient care from such textbooks.

Finally, we would like to express our gratitude to our cardiology fellows and our great staff at the teaching hospitals of Emory University, especially the Atlanta Veterans Administration Medical Center's and Emory University Hospital's cardiac catheterization laboratories, for encouraging us to write this *Pocket Guide*. We would especially like to thank our families, our teachers, and colleagues for their support and encouragement. We thank Dr. Peter Block for his sage advice and comprehensive review of our *Pocket Guide*, and are especially thankful to Mr. Donn Johnson for his technical expertise with the medical illustrations. Our deep appreciation extend to Ms. Jeanne Dow for her invaluable effort with the technical preparation of the *Pocket Guide*, as well as to our publisher, Mr. Michael Crouchet, in realizing this small dream of ours.

We are hopeful that this *Pocket Guide* will fulfill its purpose and welcome suggestions to improve its educational value.

–Andro G. Kacharava, MD, PhD
Stephen D. Clements Jr., MD
A. Maziar Zafari, MD, PhD

Abbreviations

2D	two-dimensional
3D	three-dimensional
3D-RCA	three-dimensional right coronary artery
ACC	American College of Cardiology
ACLS	advanced cardiovascular life support
ACT	activated clotting time
AHA	American Heart Association
AL	Amplatz left
AMVL	anterior mitral valve leaflet
AO	aorta
AoV	aortic valve
AP	anterior posterior = PA
AR	Amplatz right
AV	atrioventricular *or* arteriovenous
AVA	aortic valve area
BP	blood pressure
BSA	body surface area
CABG	coronary artery bypass graft
CAD	coronary artery disease
Cath	catheterization
CBC	complete blood count

CI	cardiac index
CO	cardiac output
CTA	computed tomographic angiography
CVP	central venous pressure
DBP	diastolic blood pressure
ECG	electrocardiogram
EF	ejection fraction
ESC	European Society of Cardiology
Fr	French
HF	heart failure
Hgb	hemoglobin
HR	heart rate
IABP	intra-aortic balloon pump
IJ	internal jugular
IMA	internal mammary artery
INR	international normalized ratio
IVC	inferior vena cava
JL	Judkins left
JR	Judkins right
LA	left atrium *or* left atrial
LAB	laboratory
LAD	left anterior descending
LAFB	left anterior fascicular block
LAO	left anterior oblique
LBBB	left bundle branch block
LCA	left coronary artery

LCB	left coronary bypass
LCC	left coronary cusp
LCCA	left common carotid artery
LCX	left circumflex
LIMA	left internal mammary artery
LL	left lateral
LM	left main
LPA	left pulmonary artery
LPFB	left posterior fascicular block
LSA	left subclavian artery
LV	left ventricle
LVDP	left ventricular diastolic pressure
LVEDP	left ventricular end-diastolic pressure
LVEDV	left ventricular end-diastolic volume
LVEDVI	left ventricular end-diastolic volume index
LVEF	left ventricular ejection fraction
LVESV	left ventricular end-systolic volume
MAP	mean arterial pressure
MET	metabolic equivalent of task
MP	multipurpose
MV	mitral valve
MVA	mitral valve area
NCC	noncoronary cusp
NHLBI	National Heart, Lung, and Blood Institute
NS	normal saline
NSTEMI	non-ST-elevation myocardial infarction
PA	posteroanterior
PAC	premature atrial complex
PAP	pulmonary artery pressure
PAWP	pulmonary artery wedge pressure

PCI	percutaneous coronary intervention
PDA	posterior descending artery
PLV	posterior left ventricular
Pp	pericardial pressure
PSI	pounds per square inch
PT	prothrombin time
PTCA	percutaneous transluminal coronary angioplasty
PTT	partial thromboplastin time
PVC	premature ventricular complex
PVR	pulmonary vascular resistance
Qp	pulmonary blood flow
Qs	systemic blood flow
RA	right atrium *or* right atrial
RAA	right atrial appendage
RAO	right anterior oblique
RAP	right atrial pressure
RBBB	right bundle branch block
RCA	right coronary artery
RCB	right coronary bypass
RCC	right coronary cusp
RIJ	right internal jugular
RIMA	right internal mammary artery
RPA	right pulmonary artery
RV	right ventricle
RVEDP	right ventricular end-diastolic pressure
RVOT	right ventricular outflow tract
RVP	right ventricular pressure
SA	sinoatrial
SBP	systolic blood pressure
SCAI	Society of Cardiac Angiography and Intervention

STEMI	ST-elevation myocardial infarction
SV	stroke volume
SVC	superior vena cava
SVG	saphenous venous graft
SVI	stroke volume index
SVR	systemic vascular resistance
t-PA	tissue-plasminogen activator
TTE	transthoracic echocardiography
TV	tricuspid valve
VF	ventricular fibrillation
VSD	ventricular septal defect
VT	ventricular tachycardia

Video Files of Multipurpose (MP) Catheter Manipulation

This book includes video clips instructing the reader on the techniques of multipurpose (MP) catheter manipulation. For detailed descriptions see Chapter 7.

The Laws of
Dr. F. Mason Sones*

1. Be honest.
2. Nothing is good enough.
3. Find an expert.
4. Don't read (or write)—if you must write, don't use semicolons.
5. Don't calculate.
6. Don't rely on gadgets.
7. Don't watch the clock.
8. Don't repeat experiments indefinitely.
9. Concentrate on the problem.
10. Simplify the problem.
11. Make a decision.
12. Communicate.

*As observed by Dr. William Proudfit, a friend and colleague of Dr. F. Mason Sones (1918–1985), who performed the first "selective" arteriogram on October 30, 1958 at the Cleveland Clinic.[1]

In a letter to Dr. J. Willis Hurst on August 9, 1982, Sones wrote about this event:

"When the injection (aortogram) began I was horrified to see the right coronary artery become heavily opacified and realized that the catheter tip was actually inside the dominant right coronary artery.

Initially, I could feel only unbelievable relief and gratitude that we had been fortunate enough to avert a grievous disaster. During the ensuing days I began to think that this accident might point the way for the development of a technique, which was exactly what we had been seeking."[2]

References

1. Sheldon WC. F. Mason Sones, Jr. Stormy petrel of cardiology. *Clin Cardiol.* 1994;17(7):405-407.

2. Hurst JW. History of cardiac catheterization. In *Coronary arteriography and angioplasty* (Eds. King SB III, Douglas JS Jr). New York: McGraw-Hill; 1985; 6.

CHAPTER 1

A Brief History of Cardiac Catheterization

"If you want to understand anything, observe its beginning and its development."

—Aristotle

History of a Procedure

A reader who flips through the first pages of this Pocket Guide might ask, "Do I really have to read this chapter to learn how to perform cardiac catheterization?" The rational answer is, "No." Nonetheless, please be irrational; do not skip these pages. You will be able to review the fascinating story of human curiosity, courage, and dedication of physicians and scientists who pursued their work despite the prevailing clinical and scientific dogmas to set the stage for a new generation of investigators who moved the field from diagnostic to therapeutic procedures.

No one can accurately pinpoint the exact time when humans started to be interested in cannulating blood vessels and cardiac chambers, but it is known that ancient Egyptians, Greeks, and Romans were forming tubes from hollow reeds, palm leaves, and pipes to study the function of cardiac valves in cadavers.[1] Many centuries later in 1733, British physiologist Stephen Hales performed the first catheterization of the arterial blood vessel in a horse using brass pipes and a glass tube.[2] In 1844, French physiologist Claude Bernard was first to catheterize the left and right ventricles in animals by inserting a mercury thermometer into the carotid artery and jugular vein.[3] Adolph Fick came up with a brilliant one-page note on the calculation of blood flow in 1870, which opened the experimental era of cardiac metabolism.[4] Finally, in Eberswalde, Germany in 1929, Werner Forssmann self-cannulated his antecubital vein and guided a urological catheter into his right atrium documenting its location via chest x-ray.[5] In 1941, Andre Cournand and Dickinson Richards began to utilize right heart catheterization to study cardiac output, and in 1956 they shared the Nobel Prize in Physiology and Medicine with Forssmann.

Lewis Dexter discovered in 1948 that by wedging the catheter into a distal branch of a pulmonary artery, it is feasible to record the height of the left atrial pressure.[6] In the late 1960s, Jeremy Swan and William Ganz used a balloon-tipped flow-directed catheter in the right heart to continuously measure and monitor hemodynamic tracings.[7] Ganz improved the catheter design by adding the ability to measure cardiac output using the thermodilution method. Henry Zimmerman, working at the Cleveland Clinic, is credited with combined right and left heart catheterization in 1947.[8] In 1952, Sven-Ivar Seldinger from Sweden came up with a simple and brilliant idea of over the wire insertion of a catheter, which revolutionized the approach for cannulation of arteries and veins.[9] In 1958, Mason Sones at the Cleveland Clinic developed a selective technique to cannulate coronary arteries.[10] In 1966, Melvin Judkins introduced his method for transfemoral selective coronary arteriography and subsequently popularized his first pre-formed left and right coronary catheters to simplify the process of selective cannulation of each coronary ostium.[11] Kurt Amplatz developed his own pre-formed coronary catheters in 1967.[12] In the late 1960s, Fred Schoonmaker and Spencer King introduced a single-catheter technique with a modified Sones-type catheter and published results of its use in 1974.[13]

In 1964, Charles Dotter and Melvin Judkins treated obstructed atherosclerotic peripheral arteries by using coaxial catheters to dilate their lumen to the size of 12- to 14-French (Fr) catheters.[14] In 1973, Werner Porstmann[15] and Eberhard Zeitler[16] independently published data of using a balloon technique to dilate a blood vessel, but it was Andreas Roland Gruentzig who successfully performed the first percutaneous coronary balloon angioplasty in 1977 in a 38-year-old man with an 85% stenosis in the mid segment of the left anterior descending coronary artery, thus opening the door to the fascinating era of interventional cardiology.[17]

References

1. Miller SW. *Cardiac angiography.* Boston, MA: Little, Brown; 1984.
2. Hales S. *Statistical essays, containing haemastaticks.* Vol 2. London: W Innys, R Manby, T Woodward; 1733.
3. Cournand AF. Cardiac catheterization: development of the technique its contributions to experimental medicine, and its initial applications in man. *Acta Med Scand.* 1975;579(suppl):7-32.
4. Fick A. Über die Messung des Blutquantums in den Herzventrikeln. Sitzungsber. *Phys-Med Ges Würzburg;* 1870.
5. Forssmann W. Die Sondierung des rechten Herzens. *Klin Wschr.* 1929;8:2085-2087.
6. Dexter L, Hayes FW, Burwell CS, Eppinger EC, Sagerson RP, Evans JM. Studies of congenital heart disease: II. The pressure and oxygen content of blood in the right auricle, right ventricle, and pulmonary artery in control patients, with observations on the oxygen saturation and source of pulmonary 'capillary' blood. *J Clin Invest.* 1947;26:554-560.
7. Swan HJC, Ganz W, Forrester J, Marcus H, Diamond G, Chonette D. Catheterization of the heart in man with use of a flow directed balloon-tipped catheter. *N Engl J Med.* 1970;283:447-451.
8. Zimmerman HA, Scott RW, Becker NO. Catheterization of the left side of the heart in man. *Circulation.* 1950;1:357-359.
9. Seldinger SI. Catheter replacement of the needle in percutaneous arteriography: a new technique. *Acta Radiol.* 1953;39:368-376.
10. Sones FM Jr., Shirey EK, Proudfit WL, Westcott RN. Cine-coronary arteriography (Abstract). *Circulation.* 1959;20:773.
11. Judkins MP. Selective coronary arteriography: a percutaneous transfemoral technique. *Radiology.* 1967;89:815-824.
12. Wilson WJ, Lee GB, Amplatz K. Biplane selective coronary arteriography via percutaneous transfemoral approach. *Am J Roentgenol.* 1967;100:332-340.
13. Schoonmaker FW, King SB. Coronary arteriography by the single catheter percutaneous femoral technique. Experience in 6800 cases. *Circulation.* 1974;50:735-740.
14. Dotter CT, Judkins MP. Transluminal treatment of arteriosclerotic obstruction: description of a new technique and a preliminary report of its application. *Circulation.* 1964;30:654-670.
15. Porstmann W. Ein neuer Korsett-Ballonkatheter zur transluminalen Rekanalisation nach Dotter unter besonderer Berücksichtigung von Obliterationen an den Beckenarterien. *Radio Diagn.* 1973;14:239-244.
16. Zeitler E. Percutaneous treatment of arterial blood circulation disorders of the extremities using a catheter. *Radiologe.* 1973;13(8):319-324.
17. Gruentzig A. Transluminal dilatation of coronary-artery stenosis [Letter]. *Lancet.* 1978;1:263.

CHAPTER 2

The Cardiac Catheterization Laboratory

"Any sufficiently advanced technology is indistinguishable from magic."

—Arthur C. Clarke

Catheterization Laboratory Equipment

Most cardiac catheterization laboratories consist of two separate rooms. The control room is used for monitoring the patient's vital signs, hemodynamics, and ECG tracings. Here, physicians discuss the planned procedure and write the final report. Next to the control room is the main laboratory (Figure 2.1).

The examination table can be ground-mounted or suspended from the ceiling at one end; it is movable and can be panned, raised, or lowered. The table is centered between a C-shaped structure called a gantry, which houses the laboratory's radiographic equipment. At the bottom of the gantry is the x-ray source, composed of both an x-ray generator and an x-ray tube. At the top of the gantry, or C-arm, there is an "eye-eye," the flat detector that provides high-resolution digital imagery. Other equipment located throughout the lab may include, but is not limited to, the following important items: an intra-aortic balloon pump and a code or "crash" cart with a defibrillator. In the catheterization laboratory, invasive blood pressure is monitored, and pressure waves created by cardiac

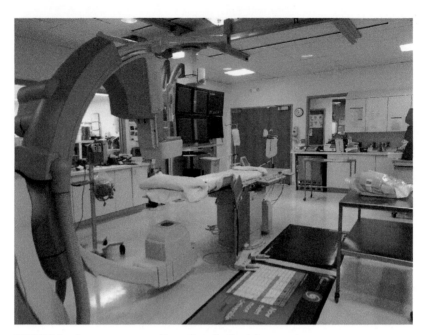

FIGURE 2.1   A contemporary cardiac catheterization laboratory.

contractions are transmitted through a fluid-filled tube connected to a pressure transducer, which converts the actual pressure waveforms into electrical signals displayed on monitors. One other piece of equipment is the power injector, which allows the physician to administer contrast rapidly and in large volumes.

The catheterization laboratory team is composed of several key positions. First, the monitoring person who in the control room closely monitors the procedure, continuously documents vital signs, ECG, hemodynamic parameters of the patient, and informs the operator of any abnormalities noticed. This position is staffed by a nurse or by a catheterization laboratory/radiology technician who is knowledgeable in cardiac hemodynamics and ECG readings. The next position is a circulating nurse who monitors O_2 saturation, CO_2 content, and noninvasive blood pressure. The circulating nurse also assists the patient and administers medications and intravenous fluids throughout the case. The other individual is the scrub person, staffed by a certified cardiovascular technician or a trained cardiovascular nurse. The role of the scrub person is to provide direct procedural assistance to the physician by panning the table, injecting contrast, and administering intra-coronary drugs.

Contrast Agents

Contrast media are used in the cardiac catheterization laboratory for intravascular and intracardiac imaging. They are available in two forms, ionic and non-ionic, categorized by their chemical makeup and differences in osmolality and viscosity. Although high viscosity is a quality of many contrast media at room temperature, viscosity decreases markedly when the medium is warmed to 37°C. The first generation of contrast agents were ionic monomers, high-osmolar, up to 1800 mOsmol/kg; the second-generation agents were non-ionic monomers with osmolality up to 850 mOsmol/kg, so called "low-osmolality" agents; and finally, the third-generation are iso-osmolar agents with osmolality less than 300 mOsmol/kg.[1] Contrast media contain iodine; because iodine is an effective x-ray absorber, contrast media are x-ray dense. All contrast agents are derived from benzoic acid. It was discovered that binding the iodine atoms to a benzene ring would enable otherwise toxic and lethal amounts of iodine to be introduced into the body and be entirely filtered by the kidneys. Contrast-induced acute kidney injury is the most significant chemotoxic event of contrast media.[2] Other chemotoxic events include nausea, vomiting, flushing, and pain during the injection.[1] High contrast volumes (> 100 mL) are associated with increased risk of developing contrast-induced nephropathy, but even small (less than 50 mL) volumes of contrast media used in high-risk patients can lead to acute renal failure requiring dialysis. Idiosyncratic reactions to contrast media such as urticaria, hives, angioedema, hypotension, coronary spasm, and bronchospasm are secondary to the release of vasoactive mediators.[1] Such anaphylactoid reactions occur in 0.05%–0.1% of patients undergoing contrast-based imaging and are independent of the dose or the iodine concentration of the contrast media. In general, a history of asthma, bronchospasm, or general atopy increases the risk for allergic reactions. In addition to anaphylactoid and chemotoxic reactions, contrast media have been shown to affect hemodynamic parameters such as heart rate, blood pressure, left ventricular pressure, and stroke volume.[1] High-osmolar ionic contrast agents decrease systolic and diastolic blood pressure, depress myocardial contractility, and increase blood volume. These agents also cause more injection-associated pain and heat sensation compared to iso-osmolar contrast agents. The knowledge of contrast media allows a cardiologist to "personalize" the type of agent used and decrease contrast-associated risk.

Radiation Exposure and Safety

Operations within the catheterization laboratory cannot take place without exposure to radiation. The x-ray beam is produced by the x-ray generator when electrons are accelerated and brought to a halt. Kilovolt levels determine the quality of x-rays produced. The quality of x-rays goes on to define the density of tissue that can be penetrated. The Joint Commission on the Accreditation of Healthcare Organizations (JCAHO) has identified peak skin dose, the maximum dose received by any local area of a patient's skin, from fluoroscopic guided procedure above 15 Gray as a sentinel event in the United States.[3] When using cineangiography, the x-ray beam is directed up from the x-ray tube beneath the table. This beam passes through the patient and is captured by the image intensifier at the top of the gantry. Radiation travels in a straight line until interacting with another object. This interaction will alter the course and quality of the beam. Misdirected radiation is called scatter to which the staff is subjected. Radiation scatter can be measured, monitored, and in fact controlled, knowing that it is highest and most dangerous when oblique angles are used during cineangiography. Additionally, it should be remembered that fluoroangiography only generates about one-fourth of the radiation of cineangiography. Fluoroscopy time for adult coronary angiography is between 10–20 minutes on average. Exposure during cinefluorography depends on the radiation dose per frame and the length of imaging time.

Without radiation safety measures in place, the amount of radiation the staff receives on a daily basis could be harmful.[4] Each laboratory must follow the standards for radiation guidelines set up by the Society for Cardiac Angiography and Intervention (SCAI). Radiation reduction involves the three classic parameters of shielding, time and distance (Table 2.1).[5]

Acrylic glass/lead shields and lead table skirts are standard safety equipment in the laboratory. These objects protect the operator from the "scatter" of the x-ray beam in addition to individual protection with lead aprons, lead eyeglasses, and thyroid shielding, which should be checked annually with fluoroscopy to detect possible cracks. Time of radiation exposure can be reduced by reducing

TABLE 2.1   Radiation reduction strategies.

For a patient and an operator:
1. Use radiation only when needed.
2. Limit use of cine, magnification modes, and high frame rates.
3. Limit use of sharp angles of x-ray beam and reduce distance to the image receptor.
4. Maximize use of collimator and monitor radiation dose in real time.

Specifically for a patient:
1. Keep table height as high as possible and patient's limbs out of the beam.
2. Change the beam angle to avoid exposure to any one skin area.

Specifically for an operator:
1. Maximize your distance from the x-ray source and patient.
2. Keep upper and lower shields in optimal position.
3. Avoid being in the field of view at all times.
4. Use appropriately maintained protective garments.

fluoroscopy time, especially by using short bursts of fluoroscopy rather than prolonged and continuous exposure. Finally, the x-ray beam is inversely proportional to the square of the distance between the subject and the source. The amount of scatter produced is directly related to the quantity and quality of the true, unaltered x-ray beam and the density of the tissue through which it passes, in addition to the total time of exposure. With proper fluoroscopic equipment, a typical cardiac angiographic study using 10 minutes of fluoroscopy and 1 minute of cinefluorography (total exposure of ≈ 7 mSv) is widely regarded as safe.[6] Average background radiation exposure per year for a member of the U.S. population is ≈ 3 mSv. Primary operators performing 10 diagnostic procedures will receive a cumulative radiation dose equivalent to 1 to 3 chest x-rays. A busy interventional cardiologist using proper technique and protection receives 2–4 mSv/year. The radiation dose can be minimized by decreasing fluoroscopy time (15% of the total fluoroscopy time occurs when the operator is not viewing an image), by placing the image intensifier closer to the patient, avoiding excessively steep angles, avoiding dense tissues in the abdomen and spine, opening the iris on the television camera, allowing a lower increase in beam intensity, and using flat panel detectors, which have more sophisticated controls. In addition, avoiding excess number of views, performing at the lowest possible frame rates, and taking fewer magnified views are strongly recommended.[4,6] Additional procedures, including left ventriculography or aortography, should be avoided if the relevant information can be acquired by noninvasive imaging modalities. The official recommendation is to wear two radiation badges during all cardiac catheterization procedures, with the second badge placed under the protective apron at the waist in order to be able to measure individual radiation exposure. If a single badge is worn, it should be on the thyroid collar.

References

1. Pasternak JJ, Williamson EE. Clinical pharmacology, uses, and adverse reactions of iodinated contrast agents: a primer for the non-radiologist. *Mayo Clin Proc.* 2012;87(4):390-402.

2. Seeliger E, Sendeski M, Rihal CS, Persson PB. Contrast-induced kidney injury: mechanisms, risk factors, and prevention. *Eur Heart J.* 2012;33(16):2007-2015.

3. Sentinel Event Policy and Procedures. http://www.jointcommission.org/ Sentinel_Event_Policy_and_Procedures/.

4. Best PJ, Skelding KA, Mehran R, et al. SCAI consensus document on occupational radiation exposure to the pregnant cardiologist and technical personnel. *Catheter Cardiovasc Interv.* 2011;77(2):232-241.

5. Chambers CE, Fetterly KA, Holzer R, et al. Radiation safety program for the cardiac catheterization laboratory. *Catheter Cardiovasc Interv.* 2011;77(4):546-556.

6. Fazel R, Gerber TC, Balter S, et al. Approaches to enhancing radiation safety in cardiovascular imaging: a scientific statement from the American Heart Association. *Circulation.* 2014;130(19):1730-1748.

CHAPTER 3

The Tools

"One who knows strengths and weaknesses of different tools lowers the risk and succeeds often."

—Anonymous

Percutaneous Access Needles

There are two major types of access needle design: the standard disposable Seldinger needle and the standard direct front-wall needle. A standard Seldinger-type access needle has a blunted bevel and is accompanied by a stylet. A standard direct front-wall needle has a sharper bevel angle and does not have the second component such as a stylet. It may or may not have a baseplate hub (Figure 3.1).

The 18-gauge, 0.049-inch diameter needle, up to 3 inches in length, allows passage of a flexible 0.035-inch guidewire with a 3 mm "J" tip. The major advantage of the direct front-wall needle is the ability to decrease the risk of site bleeding and hematoma formation as a result of posterior vessel wall puncture. This is a major advantage when cardiac catheterization is performed in a fully anti-coagulated patient. A direct front-wall needle attached to a 12-mL syringe is used when attempting to establish central venous access. In situations such as a small, calcified, tortuous femoral vessel or the use of an anticoagulant, a smaller needle may be preferred to reduce the risk of access complications. The Micropuncture Kit (Cook Medical, Inc., Bloomington, IN) includes a 21-gauge needle and a 4-Fr (1 Fr is 0.33 mm) sheath (Figure 3.2).

Although the smaller needle reduces the size of the arterial hole by more than 50%, there is no clear evidence that the Micropuncture Kit reduces vascular complications.[1,2] In high-risk procedures with

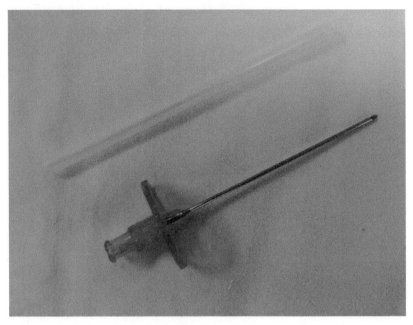

FIGURE 3.1 A standard direct front-wall needle (Cook Medical, Inc.) has a sharper bevel angle than the Seldinger-type needle (not shown).

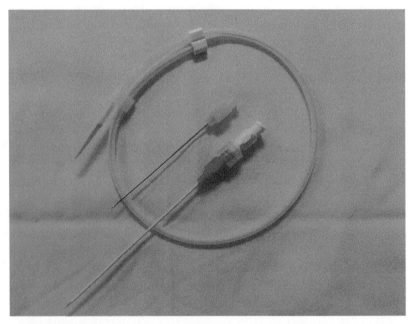

FIGURE 3.2 The Micropuncture Kit (Angiodynamics Inc., Cambridge, UK) with a 21-gauge needle and a 4-Fr sheath is shown.

difficult single arterial or venous access, percutaneous access can be achieved by a specific ultrasound-guided needle.[3,4]

Guidewires

The guidewire is the cornerstone of Seldinger's idea of percutaneous access of the blood vessel.[5] Basic guidewires differ in shape (straight versus J-tipped), diameter, length, and structure. Most invasive cardiologists use flexible 0.035- or 0.038-inch J-tip guidewires when obtaining vascular access since it decreases the risk of vessel dissection (Figure 3.3).

The 0.021- or 0.025-inch straight-tip guidewires are used primarily when obtaining radial arterial access, or when attempting to stiffen the balloon-tipped pulmonary artery catheter. The straight, soft-tipped wires are used in crossing severely stenosed aortic valves. The decision on length of the guidewire, short (30–45 cm) versus long (120–150 cm), is made based on the type and length of the sheath to be placed. The extra-long guidewires' (250–300 cm) primary use is to avoid repeatedly negotiating and crossing

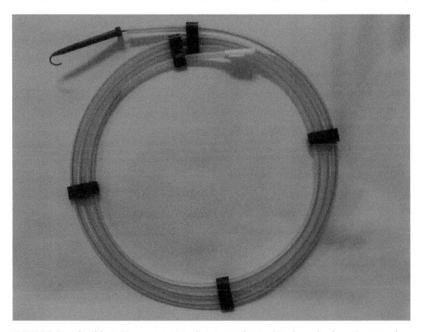

FIGURE 3.3   Flexible 0.035- or 0.038-inch J-tip guidewire (Cook Medical, Inc.) are used to decrease the risk of vessel dissection.

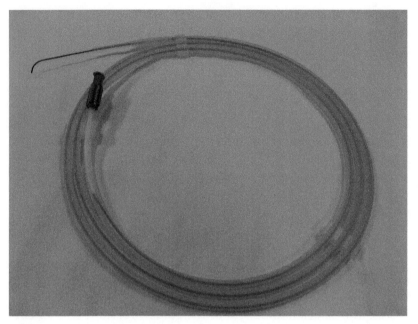

FIGURE 3.4   The Zipwire (Boston Scientific Inc., Chaska, MN) is a "slippery" hydrophilic guidewire.

tortuous and/or diseased vessels during the catheter exchange process. The general structure of most guidewires is similar: a flexible, distal spring coil, a regular or gradually tapered, movable central core, usually made from stainless steel, and an external hydrophilic coating to decrease thrombogenicity and friction. In order to navigate through the severely diseased and/or tortuous peripheral blood vessels, a Zipwire—a specific "slippery" hydrophilic guidewire with good steerability and torque response—is used (Figure 3.4).

Some operators use a stopcock device, locked at the distal end of the wire, to improve handling and maneuvering of these wires. The use of "slippery" wires when obtaining vascular access is not recommended due to the potential for the wire to slip through the access needle and be lost in the circulation. In addition, there is a potential problem with shearing off the polyurethane cover of the slippery wire by the tip of the access needle.

Vascular Sheaths and Dilators

Vascular sheaths are major elements of a cardiac catheterization procedure (Figure 3.5).[6]

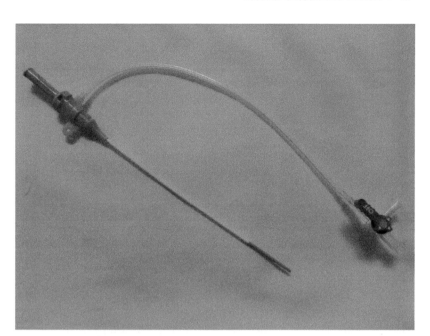

FIGURE 3.5   Terumo Pinnacle Sheath (Terumo Medical, Elkton, MD) is one type of vascular sheath used in cardiac catheterization.

In general, all vascular sheaths have removable, stiff dilators made from Teflon or polyethylene. These dilators have a common structure that includes a side arm with a three-way stopcock and a back-bleed protection valve/membrane, but they differ in length, diameter, and stiffness. The side arm's three-way stopcock can be used for aspiration of blood, flushing of the sheath, medication injections and pressure monitoring. The structure of the back-bleed protection valve/membrane is important since tight valves create problems with rotations of the catheter; on the other hand, loose valves lead to back-bleeding.

When dealing with a tight valve, the operator should moisten the catheter with wet gauze frequently. The decision of what sheath type to use is based on the patient's medical history and the purpose of the procedure. Traditionally, 4- to 6-Fr sheaths are used for diagnostic cardiac catheterization. It is important to remember that after placing the sheath, it can be changed and upgraded to a higher-diameter sheath if needed. Sheath length varies from short (6 cm) to long (45 cm). In general, longer sheaths are used to prevent vascular spasm in case of radial artery access or to straighten tortuous ileofemoral vessels and improve torque control over the diagnostic catheter. Certain types of sheaths have higher resistance to kinking and could potentially decrease the risk of vessel trauma in very tortuous vessels or during a change of a patient's position if required. Another useful type of sheath, used to allow access to calcified vessel walls and Dacron artificial grafts, is a Terumo pinnacle sheath with a smooth transition from a dilator to a sheath (Figure 3.5).

Catheters

Catheters vary in structure, diameter, length, configuration, and in the presence or absence of side holes.[6] For simplicity, the entire pool of catheters can be divided in two large groups: those used for "right heart" catheterization and those used for "left heart" catheterization. The *right heart catheters* can be further subdivided into two groups: catheters with and without balloon-tipped flow-direction. Most of the balloon-tipped, flow-directed catheters have a latex balloon at the distal end of the catheter, which can be inflated to a volume of approximately 2 mL as the catheter tip advances beyond the sheath during catheterization. A balloon-tipped, flow-directed, dual-lumen thermodilution Swan-Ganz catheter is used to determine cardiac output by the thermodilution method (Figure 3.6).[7] This catheter has multiple lumens for distal and proximal pressure measurement and a thermistor located about 4 cm from the distal tip. The proximal port is also used for the injection of an indicator (cold saline in most cases). Two additional lumens with side ports permit placement of right atrial and right ventricular pacing wires for pacing.

The Berman balloon-tipped, flow-directed angiographic catheter does not have the end hole but has multiple side holes to prevent recoil during pressure injection of the contrast agent (Figure 3.7).

The single-hole multipurpose catheter does not have a balloon tip and is used for blood sampling and pressure monitoring during right heart catheterization. The Grollman pigtail angiography catheter has an angled tip, which is formed to ease access to the pulmonary artery and perform pulmonary angiography (Figure 3.8).

Angiographic catheters with multiple side holes provide stable, high-flow injection of the contrast agent and are utilized for ventriculography and large-vessel angiography. Pigtail catheters (6-Fr,

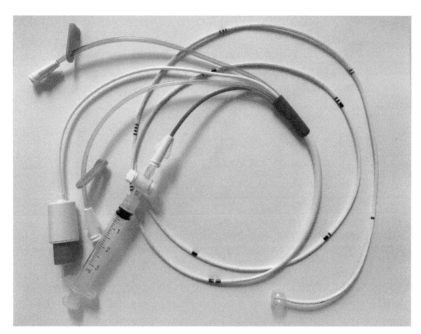

FIGURE 3.6   A balloon-tipped, flow-directed, dual-lumen thermodilution Swan-Ganz catheter (Arrow International, Inc., Reading, PA) has multiple lumens for distal and proximal pressure measurement and a thermistor located about 4 cm from the distal tip.

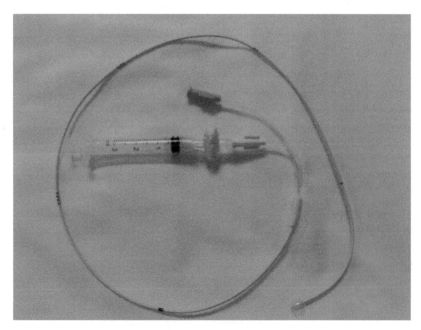

FIGURE 3.7   The Berman balloon-tipped, flow-directed angiographic catheter (Arrow International, Inc.) has multiple side holes to prevent recoil.

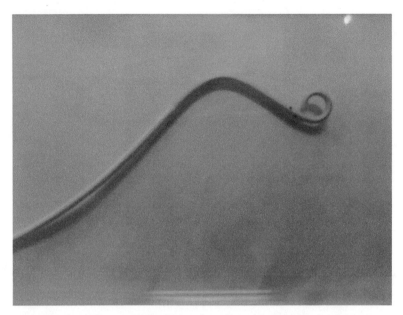

FIGURE 3.8   The Grollman pigtail angiography catheter (Cordis Medical, Johnson & Johnson, Miami Lakes, FL) has an angled tip to ease access to the pulmonary artery.

110-cm length; Figure 3.9) have a curled tip, with either a straight or angled distal segment and 4 or 6 side holes and an end hole. The angled pigtail catheter is usually used in left ventriculography, and the straight pigtail catheter for aortography. Other angiographic catheters—e.g., Schoonmaker-King multipurpose (2 side holes and an end hole) or NIH (2 or 4 side holes without an end hole)—are easily maneuverable, and useful when brachial or radial approaches are utilized for left ventriculography (Figure 3.9).

Diagnostic coronary angiography catheters come in different lengths (80–125 cm), external diameters (4- to 6-Fr), curve shapes (primary, secondary, and tertiary), arm lengths (3.7–6.2 cm, JL 3.5 to JL 6, respectively) and can be broadly classified into two major groups: preformed catheters (Judkins, Amplatz, Tiger, and coronary bypass) (Figure 3.10, A-C) and unformed catheters (Sones, Schoonmaker-King) (Figure 3.11).

The principal advantage of all preformed catheters is easy access to the normally located ostia of the native coronary vessels or bypass grafts. These catheters require less dexterity and provide a steeper learning curve. Using unformed and multipurpose catheters (Sones, Schoonmaker-King) requires more experience and dexterity, as described in detail in Chapter 7.

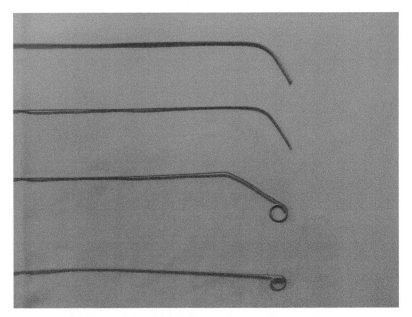

FIGURE 3.9   Easily maneuverable catheters that are useful when brachial or radial approaches are utilized for left ventriculography include the NIH (**top**), multipurpose (**second from top**), angled pigtail (**third from top**), and straight pigtail (**bottom**) catheters (Cordis Corp., Johnson & Johnson).

The number of catheter exchanges directly correlates with the risk of thromboembolic complications. When the operator has mastered the multipurpose catheter, he/she will be able to use a single catheter, avoiding multiple catheter exchanges over the wire in order to cannulate the left and right coronary arteries and all bypass grafts (except for the mammary graft), as well as perform pressure measurement and left ventriculography. The final choice of the catheter depends on patient safety, operator's experience, site of access, and knowledge of coronary and bypass graft anatomy.

Manifold

This crucial, plastic device is an indispensable part of any cardiac catheterization procedure (Figure 3.12). Types of manifold systems vary, but the major purposes of the device are to provide adequate connection to a pressure monitoring system with normal

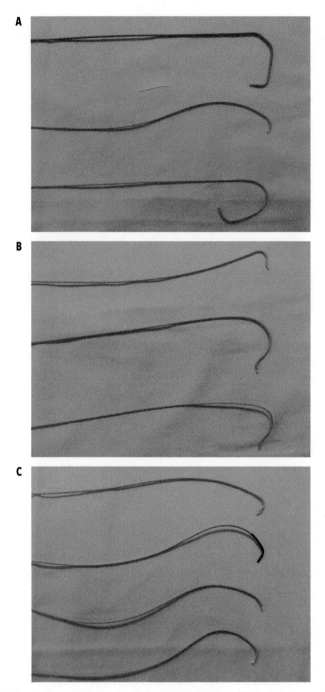

FIGURE 3.10   Preformed catheters include: (**A**) Tiger (Terumo Medical, Somerset, NJ), Judkins right and Judkins left; (**B**) modified right and left Amplatz; (**C**) IMA and COBRA coronary bypass right and left, (Cordis Corp., Johnson & Johnson).

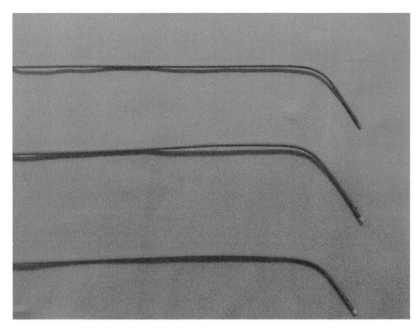

FIGURE 3.11   Use of multipurpose catheters (Schoonmaker-King, Sones 2 and 1) (Cordis Corp., Johnson & Johnson) requires more experience and dexterity.

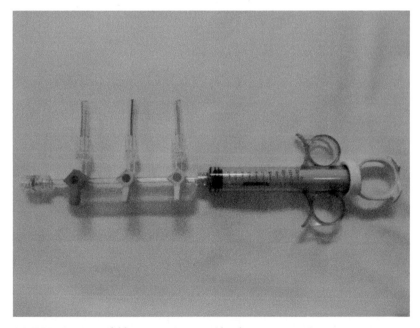

FIGURE 3.12   A manifold's purpose is to provide adequate connection to a pressure monitoring system with normal saline flush and contrast agent solutions. This manifold is connected to a 12-mL syringe (CPT Medical Inc., Easley, SC).

saline flush and contrast agent solutions. In order to accomplish these functions, the manifold is designed to have 3 or 4 stopcocks attached. The first stopcock is hooked to a pressure transducer, the second one to normal saline, and the third stopcock is connected to the contrast agent. The fourth stopcock is used in variable fashion: Some operators connect it to a container where discarded fluid can be placed; others attach a 5 mL syringe filled with 100 mcg/mL of nitroglycerin solution, which can be used as needed for intracoronary injection during coronary angiography.[8] This eliminates the need to disconnect and reconnect the injector syringe from the manifold for pre- and post-intracoronary nitroglycerine injections.

The distal port of the manifold is used to connect to either the catheter or the side port of the vascular sheath. The proximal port of the manifold is connected to a 10- to 12-mL syringe.

References

1. Ambrose JA, Lardizabal J, Mouanoutoua M, et al. Femoral micropuncture or routine introducer study (FEMORIS). *Cardiology.* 2014;129(1):39-43.

2. Pradhan A, Abbott JD. Improvements in transfemoral catheterization access techniques. *Cardiology.* 2014;129(1):36-38.

3. Byrne RA, Cassese S, Linhardt M, Kastrati A. Vascular access and closure in coronary angiography and percutaneous intervention. *Nat Rev Cardiol.* 2013;10(1):27-40.

4. Sheth RA, Walker TG, Saad WE, et al. Quality improvement guidelines for vascular access and closure device use. *J Vasc Interv Radiol.* 2014;25(1):73-84.

5. Seldinger SI. Catheter replacement of the needle in percutaneous arteriography: a new technique. *Acta Radiol.* 1953;39:368-376.

6. Casserly IP, Messenger JC. Technique and catheters. *Cardiol Clin.* 2009;27:417-432.

7. Chatterjee K. The Swan-Ganz catheters: past, present, and future. A viewpoint. *Circulation.* 2009;119:147-152.

8. Howard B, Kacharava AG. Proposal of manifold variation for use during cardiac catheterization. *Cath Lab Digest.* 2013;21(4):2.

CHAPTER 4

Precatheterization Care

"Diligence is the mother of good fortune."

—Benjamin Disraeli

The Rule of the Rules

A meticulous preprocedural work-up keeps major and minor complications of cardiac catheterization at a minimum.[1,2] First, the referring physician provides the indication for the type of invasive procedure requested and is available for questions. Second, the invasive cardiologist performing the procedure has a solid knowledge base of (1) general indications and contraindications of the requested procedure, (2) methods of controlling pre- and postprocedural risk factors, and (3) types of possible procedural difficulties and complications and how to handle these. Third, the operator follows the unwritten rule that time spent examining and evaluating a patient, studying the paper chart or electronic medical record, reviewing previous coronary angiography images and pressure tracings (Box), and documenting findings is rewarded by procedural safety and patient satisfaction.

An invasive cardiologist should never hesitate to:

1. Postpone an elective procedure if important data are missing during the preprocedural assessment.
2. Ask for advice or help from a colleague when needed at any step of the procedure.
3. Cancel the procedure if it is not indicated, and discuss the case with the referring physicians.

The standard set of laboratory data—complete blood count (CBC), serum electrolytes, serum creatinine, and anticoagulation parameters (PT/PTT/INR)—should be obtained, reviewed,

The Rules of Reading Coronary Angiography Images and Pressure Tracings

1. Note the artificial devices (pacemakers, wires, pacemaker/ defibrillator leads, sternal wires, prosthetic valves) and amount of calcification (vascular, pericardial, valvular, annular) on cardiac fluorography.
2. Determine the catheter type and its French size to estimate the size of coronary vessels.
3. Determine the view:
   a. Find the spine: if on the left side of the screen, view is right anterior oblique (RAO); if on the right side of the screen, view is left anterior oblique (LAO); if in the middle, view is posterior anterior (PA).
   b. If spine is not visible, find the ascending portion of the catheter: if on the left side of the screen, view is RAO; if on the right side of the screen, view is LAO; if in the middle, view is PA.
   c. If spine and ascending portion of the catheter cannot be seen clearly, note the orientation of the ribs on the screen: if from left to right, view is RAO; if from right to left, view is LAO.
   d. If spine and ascending portion of the catheter cannot be seen clearly, look at the distal segment of the catheter: if the tip of the catheter crosses well over the ascending portion of the catheter, the view is RAO; if it comes near or just touches the ascending portion of the catheter, the view is PA; and if it is away from the ascending portion of the catheter, forming what can be described as "a wide-open fisherman's hook," the view is LAO.
   e. If the sternum is visualized on the extreme left of the screen, the view is left lateral.
   f. To determine cranial or caudal orientation of the view, look at the amount of diaphragm on the screen: if a significant portion of diaphragm can be seen at view initiation, this view has cranial angulation, and if not, it has caudal angulation. If this rule is not helpful, look at the vessels best seen on the view: when the left circumflex artery is coming down and is well outlined together with obtuse marginal branches without overlapping

the other vessels, the view is with caudal angulation. On the contrary, when the left anterior descending artery and diagonals are well outlined and the left circumflex is directed up and not well visualized due to overlap, the view is with cranial angulation.

g. In regard to right coronary, the view with cranial angulation gives the best visualization of the crux and the distal right coronary artery with posterior descending artery bifurcation. Caudal angulation rarely is used in routine diagnostic coronary angiography of the RCA.

4. When determining the severity of stenosis, assess all the views and compare them to an adjacent reference segment that is normal-appearing on angiography and to the catheter size. Eccentric stenosis may appear normal in one or two views. Review and describe the lesion: its complexity, presence of calcification, dissection, and thrombus. Comment on location and length of the lesion. Also comment on extent and pattern of luminal irregularities, dynamic changes of epicardial blood vessels caused by spasm, and myocardial bridging. Describe flow pattern and runoff of the contrast. Note source, destination, and magnitude of collaterals and presence of abnormal communications such as arteriovenous and arteriocameral fistulas.

5. Use available hemodynamic data in addition to angiographic data when judging the severity of ostial coronary stenosis.

6. Compare with previous angiographic studies if available.

7. Identify the cardiac rhythm, note recording speed and pressure scale, and time the pressure tracings based on simultaneous ECG strips.

8. Always interpret the hemodynamic waveforms in conjunction with the patient's clinical presentation.

and corrected if possible. All patients should have a solid, secure, 21-gauge intravenous access and preprocedure ECG. Patients with diabetes mellitus on long-acting insulin therapy should administer half of the evening dose of insulin and hold the morning dose, with blood glucose levels frequently monitored and appropriately controlled with short-acting insulin. Oral hypoglycemic medications should be placed on hold on the day of cardiac catheterization until feeding is resumed postprocedure. It is recommended to hydrate patients 4–6 hours pre- and 4–6 hours postprocedure with 0.45% or 0.9% normal saline. Also, patients should discontinue use of nonsteroidal anti-inflammatory drugs and, if possible, diuretics and ACE inhibitors on procedure day. It may be prudent to hold beta-blockers preprocedure in patients with previous history of anaphylactic reaction to contrast dye (in case epinephrine is needed to treat recurrent anaphylaxis). Antibiotic prophylaxis is not routinely indicated, but in rare cases when prophylaxis is considered, selection of the antibiotic agent should be based on its efficacy against the most common skin pathogens, and it should be given 30–60 minutes before the procedure. If fluoroquinolones or vancomycin is chosen, the agent should be given 2 hours before the procedure.

Fourth, it is an *absolute contraindication* to proceed without the patient's signed informed consent. The planned procedure should be explained to a patient in terms that are easy to understand, risks and benefits clearly outlined, and all questions related to the procedure appropriately answered via the process of informed consent. The informed consent form should be signed by a patient who has been 24 hours free from any form of sedation. If a patient is unable to sign the consent, it should be obtained from a person who has durable power of attorney regarding the patient's health.

Fifth, after the above steps are completed, the optimal step-by-step plan for a scheduled procedure should be shared with the cardiac catheterization laboratory team participating in the procedure. Preprocedure note and orders should be written prior to the start of the procedure.

WHAT IF AN OPERATOR ENCOUNTERS ONE OF THE FOLLOWING PROBLEMS?

Reaction to Sedatives Used in the Cardiac Catheterization Laboratory

The commonly used combination of medications is midazolam and fentanyl given intravenously. These drugs are short-acting, titratable, and have reversal agents. The rapid onset allows observation of the sedative effect before administration of additional doses. Fentanyl causes the least amount of histamine release when compared with other opioids and is less likely to cause hypotension after injection. Cardiovascular effects of midazolam are minimal at sedative doses. The key point in prevention of oversedation and respiratory depression is the judicious use of medications with meticulous patient monitoring (vital signs, pulse oximetry, and capnography), especially in older patients. Lack of patient's response to verbal stimuli is often a sign of impending respiratory depression. At the first signs of oversedation, airways should be protected, oxygen delivered in adequate amount, and reversal with 0.4 mg of naloxone and 0.4 mg of flumazenil administered intravenously, and repeated as needed. If 10 mg naloxone and 5 mg of flumazenil do not reverse the signs of oversedation, other causes should be considered. Patients who receive reversal agents should be observed for several hours to avoid resedation. Flumazenil administration may cause seizures, especially in patients who have an underlying seizure disorder or in patients with benzodiazepine dependence.

Anaphylactoid Reaction to Local Anesthetics or Contrast Dye

Local anesthetics can be subdivided into two groups: amides and esters. The amide (two "i") group includes lidocaine, bupivacaine, and ropivacaine. The ester (one "i") class consists of procaine, chloroprocaine, and tetracaine. Esters are derivatives of para-aminobenzoic acid, which is known to be allergenic. While the amide local anesthetics are not derived from the same compound, multidose vials may contain a preservative called methylparaben, which is structurally similar to para-aminobenzoic acid and may cause allergic reaction in some patients. An operator should document the presence of an allergic reaction to a specific local anesthetic and use an alternative class. If the original drug that caused a true allergic reaction is not known, it is advised to premedicate the patient with diphenhydramine and prednisone prior to the elective procedure, or in an emergent case, proceed without local anesthetic but with higher dose of opioid analgesics and benzodiazepines. As opposed to true anaphylactic reactions, which are mediated by IgE, contrast reactions appear to result from direct complement and/or mast cell activation and are categorized as anaphylactoid.[3] With this type of reaction, vasoactive substances are released from circulating basophils and tissue mast cells. The risk is highest in patients with a history of prior contrast reactions and in individuals with atopic conditions such as asthma. Such patients benefit from premedication with steroids and antihistamines, i.e., 40–60 mg oral prednisone administered at 12 hours, 6 hours, and 1 hour prior to cardiac catheterization, accompanied by 25–50 mg diphenhydramine administered 12 hours and again 1 hour prior to procedure. Use of an oral H_2-blocker administered 12 hours and 1 hour before the procedure is optional. It is a common misconception that patients allergic to shellfish are at increased risk for adverse reactions to contrast media beyond that of any atopic individual or patients with other food allergies. The association between seafood allergies and contrast reactions has been attributed to iodine; however, iodine and iodide are small molecules that typically do not cause allergic reactions. The culprit behind shellfish allergies is thought to be tropomyosin proteins, which are unrelated to iodine.[4]

The severity of allergic reactions have been classified as mild (grade I: nausea, sneezing, vertigo), usually not requiring therapy; moderate (grade II: hives, pruritus, chills, fever), treated with intravenous diphenhydramine 25–50 mg with or without ranitidine 50 mg in 20 mL normal saline over 10 min; and severe (grade III: bronchospasm, laryngospasm or edema, hypotension/shock, angioedema, occasionally hypertension, cardiac arrhythmias and pulmonary edema), treated with epinephrine 10 mcg/mL boluses (1 mL of 1:10000 solution diluted up in 9 mL of normal saline) until blood pressure response, then drip 1–4 mcg/min to maintain desired blood pressure, normal saline infusion up to 1–3 L/hour plus diphenhydramine 50–100 mg intravenously and hydrocortisone 200–400 mg intravenously, plus O_2 by mask and albuterol nebulizer, endotracheal intubation if necessary; ranitidine 50 mg in 20 mL normal saline over 10 min is optional. Grade III reaction is a devastating complication, and cardiac catheterization laboratory personnel should be familiar with the current advanced cardiac life support (ACLS) guidelines in order to tackle the problem quickly and effectively.

Other Adverse Reactions to Local Anesthetics and Contrast Dye

Overdosing of lidocaine may be accompanied by seizures in patients without a history of a seizure disorder. Chemotoxic events such as nausea and vomiting are quite common with injection of contrast, and usually are effectively addressed with antiemetics (e.g., promethazine 25–50 mg intravenously).

References

1. Sanborn TA, Tcheng JE, Anderson HV, et al. ACC/AHA/SCAI 2014 health policy statement on structured reporting for the cardiac catheterization laboratory: a report of the American College of Cardiology Clinical Quality Committee. *Circulation.* 2014;129(24):2578-2609.

2. Patel MR, Bailey SR, Bonow RO, et al. ACCF/SCAI/AATS/AHA/ASE/ASNC/ HFSA/HRS/SCCM/SCCT/SCMR/STS 2012 appropriate use criteria for diagnostic catheterization: American College of Cardiology Foundation Appropriate Use Criteria Task Force Society for Cardiovascular Angiography and Interventions American Association for Thoracic Surgery American Heart Association, American Society of Echocardiography American Society of Nuclear Cardiology Heart Failure Society of America Heart Rhythm Society, Society of Critical Care Medicine Society of Cardiovascular Computed Tomography Society for Cardiovascular Magnetic Resonance Society of Thoracic Surgeons. *Catheter Cardiovasc Interv.* 2012;80(3):E50-E81.

3. Pasternak JJ, Williamson EE. Clinical pharmacology, uses, and adverse reactions of iodinated contrast agents: a primer for the non-radiologist. *Mayo Clin Proc.* 2012;87(4):390-402.

4. Schabelman E, Witting M. The relationship of radiocontrast, iodine, and seafood allergies: a medical myth exposed. *J Emerg Med.* 2010;39(5):701-707.

CHAPTER 5

Vascular Access

"The beginning is half of everything."

—Pythagoras

Percutaneous Vascular Access

The process of planning and obtaining percutaneous vascular access follows certain rules, and these rules should be followed in order to decrease the rate of potential complications.[1-3] Three major, obligatory rules for every operator to follow are: (1) adequate knowledge of the medical history of the patient; (2) knowledge of the anatomy of the access site; and (3) focused preprocedural cardiovascular examination, with special attention on presence, strength, and quality of distal pulses, presence of bruits at arterial access sites, and presence and character of symptoms of intermittent claudication. The choice of access site depends on factors that can be divided into patient-specific and operator-preferred choices (Table 5.1).[4-6] Aortic aneurysmal disease is not an absolute contraindication to femoral access, but it is generally recommended to use brachial or radial access as an alternative.

Femoral Artery Approach

The right or left common femoral arteries are often used as vascular access sites for percutaneous diagnostic cardiac catheterization. It is recommended to avoid femoral access in patients with known, complex artificial aorto-ileo-femoral grafts, large abdominal aneurysms, and severe peripheral vascular disease. Femoral

TABLE 5.1 Advantages and disadvantages of radial, brachial, and femoral access sites for left heart catheterization and angiography.

	ADVANTAGE	DISADVANTAGE
Radial artery	• Reduced risk of bleeding • Immediate ambulation • Short hospital stay • Improved patient comfort	• Longer learning curve • Technically more difficult • Increased radiation exposure • Difficult coronary cannulation • Potential problem with subsequent use of the radial artery as a graft in CABG surgery
Brachial artery	• Reduced risk of bleeding • Immediate ambulation • Short hospital stay • Improved patient comfort	• Longer learning curve • Technically more difficult • Increased radiation exposure • Increased risk of limb ischemia
Femoral artery	• Technically easier • Easy coronary cannulation • Less radiation exposure • Left lateral projection easily obtainable • Easy access to both internal mammary arteries	• Increased risk of bleeding • Delayed ambulation • Patient discomfort

artery access should be also avoided on the side where a decreased femoral pulse is associated with auscultatory bruits and a history of intermittent claudication involving the thigh and gluteal muscles. If both right and left femoral arteries are adequate for cannulation, the right femoral artery is usually chosen as the preferred site of entry due to general convenience. Hair at an access site is removed before the procedure with electric clippers or a depilatory cream. Both inguinal areas are prepared and draped under sterile conditions. The operator identifies anatomical landmarks such as the anterior superior iliac spine and the os pubis. The inguinal ligament outlines the imaginary line connecting the above two structures in nonobese patients, and the point of maximal impulse of arterial pulsation is usually located between one-third and one-half of the distance from the medial end of the inguinal ligament (Figure 5.1). At this anticipated puncture site, an operator places the tip of the "mosquito" forceps and obtains a fluoroscopic image of the femoral head (this is especially indicated in obese patients, in whom the inguinal crease orientation may lead to a lower arterial stick). In the majority of adults, the common femoral artery bifurcates caudal to the middle of the femoral head, so the point above the middle of the femoral head and below the level of inguinal ligament is the

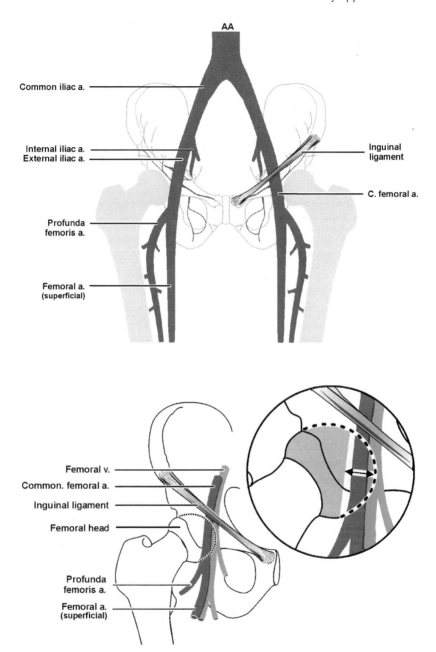

FIGURE 5.1 Anatomic relationship of blood vessels to pelvic landmarks is shown.

optimal place for puncture. The operator places the tips of the four fingers of his hand over this area in order to localize the point of maximal impulse of the arterial pulse. Further tuning is done by placing the site of the maximal arterial impulse in between the tips of the index and middle fingers of the other hand. The path of the common femoral artery is outlined by positioning the tips of the index and middle fingers, slightly spread apart perpendicular to the patient's inguinal ligament, in such a manner that the point of maximal arterial impulse is projected in the center of the imaginary line connecting the tips of those fingers.

The patient is notified that he/she might feel a needle stick accompanied by a burning sensation in the groin area, caused by the local anesthetic. Injection of the skin after localizing the site of arterial access gives the operator an opportunity to be more accurate and use less anesthetic to provide adequate local anesthesia. The skin and superficial tissue over the access site is anesthetized with a 25-gauge needle containing 5 mL of 1% warm lidocaine solution (warming the solution and mixing it with sodium bicarbonate in 10:1 proportion decreases the patient's discomfort). If the patient is slim, this is all that is needed. Otherwise, a 22-gauge needle and additional 10 mL of the anesthetic may be required. Care should be exercised in not injecting the anesthetic into the vascular structure. If a patient feels pain at the site of access at any point while the operator is attempting to obtain access, additional anesthetic is delivered locally. If the pain is extremely sharp and radiating down into the leg, no anesthetic should be injected; instead, the needle should be immediately withdrawn and repositioned medially to avoid femoral nerve damage. After the tissue is anesthetized, 2 possible approaches (with and without early subcutaneous tunnel creation) to cannulate the common femoral artery are used. The method of choice for cannulation depends on the operator's preference. A single anterior arterial wall stick should be the goal. In one method, the operator lightly holds an 18-gauge (0.049 inch in diameter), open-bore arterial access needle at the hub with the thumb and index fingers of the right hand (middle finger sometimes used to provide support for the needle), and inserts the needle at a 45-degree angle with the bevel pointed upwards through the skin above the maximum arterial impulse resting between the left index and middle fingers (Figure 5.2A). The operator considers the patient's body habitus since it will affect the horizontal distance between the skin puncture site and the arteriotomy site, with thinner patients having a significantly shorter distance in comparison

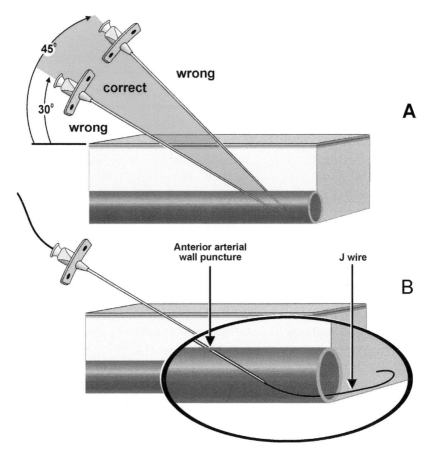

FIGURE 5.2 Correct angle of entry into the artery is shown in **Panel A** and insertion of the guidewire in **Panel B**.

to obese individuals. This distance needs to be taken into account to prevent a high stick in obese patients. As the tip of the needle is gently advanced through the subcutaneous tissue, the operator tries to feel the arterial pulsation transmitted from the anterior wall of the artery to the needle hub. Up-and-down motion of the hub suggests correct passage towards the anterior surface of the artery; the needle should be gently advanced until a strong pulsatile blood return is observed, which suggests successful entry into the arterial lumen. When this occurs, the operator should avoid advancing the tip of the needle further. Side-to-side movements of the needle hub indicate that the needle has passed medial or lateral to the artery, and the needle needs to be withdrawn. When the tip of the needle is in the lumen of the common femoral artery, the J-tip 0.035-Fr guidewire is inserted and advanced through the needle into the vessel lumen (Figure 5.2B).

The needle is removed after a small nick of the skin is made with a scalpel at the level of needle entrance in order to ease the subsequent insertion of the sheath or dilator over the guidewire into the arterial lumen by gentle rotational movement. Once the sheath is appropriately positioned, the dilator and the guidewire are removed and cleaned. Approximately 2–3 mL arterial blood is aspirated through the sheath, and the sheath is flushed with 8–10 mL normal saline. The sheath side port is then connected to the manifold for femoral artery pressure recording.

When using a micropuncture needle after the access area is properly sterilized and anesthetized, the 21-gauge needle is inserted into the common femoral artery at 45 degrees. The stick should be neither too high nor too low in relation to the femoral head. When the artery is punctured, the backflow is not as pulsatile as with the 18-gauge needle. Next, a floppy-tipped, 0.01-inch guidewire is inserted through the needle and advanced into the artery under fluoroscopic guidance. The wire should appear free and mobile to ensure that it is in the vessel lumen. If the stick height is not optimal, then the needle and wire can be easily removed. After 3 minutes of manual pressure, access can be reattempted. When the 0.01-inch floppy wire is advanced into the common iliac artery, the needle is removed. Next, a 4-Fr micropuncture sheath with a 3-Fr dilator is advanced over the wire into the femoral artery. The wire and dilator are then removed from the sheath, and a regular 0.03-inch guidewire is inserted into the micropuncture sheath and advanced into the distal aorta. The micropuncture sheath can then be replaced with a standard sheath.

Brachial Artery Approach

The right or left brachial artery can be used as access sites for percutaneous diagnostic cardiac catheterization.[7] The left brachial artery is used by operators who prefer Judkins catheters, and the right brachial artery is usually chosen by operators who are accustomed to using multipurpose catheters. With right brachial access, the operator avoids the flow path of the left carotid artery with its potential risks; it is also more convenient for an operator, and the exposure to radiation is less.

When the site of access is prepared and draped under sterile conditions, the operator palpates the distal brachial artery slightly above the antecubital fossa (point of maximal impulse is usually located 1 cm above it) (Figure 5.3). The artery is superficial and fixed at this level, which makes it easy to access and to securely compress against the humerus if needed. Further tuning can be done as described for accessing the common femoral artery. The skin and superficial tissue over the access site is anesthetized with a 25-gauge needle containing 3–5 mL of 1% warm lidocaine solution. If the patient feels pain at the site of access at any point while attempting to cannulate the brachial artery, additional anesthetic should be delivered. If the pain is extremely sharp and radiating down into the arm, no anesthetic should be injected; instead, the needle should be withdrawn immediately and repositioned laterally to avoid median nerve damage. To cannulate the brachial artery, a single anterior arterial wall stick should be made. Some operators prefer to use a micropuncture kit with a 21-gauge access needle, but the standard 18-gauge access needle can also be used. The rest of the brachial access steps are routine and described with the femoral approach. Heparin 40 units/kg bolus should be administered intravenously as soon as access is obtained and anticoagulation time (ACT) checked to keep it > 200 seconds to avoid sheath thrombosis. To prevent arterial spasm, 100–200 mcg nitroglycerine or 3.0–5.0 mg of verapamil is injected into the artery through the side port of the sheath.

Radial Artery Approach

Prior to proceeding with accessing the radial artery, the Allen test can be performed to check if the palmar arch is intact.[4] Ideally, in order to increase the validity of the test, pulse oximetry and plethysmography are utilized. The operator palpates the radial and ulnar arteries on the arm planned for the procedure. A pulse oximetry monitor is attached to the patient's index finger; wave amplitude and oxygen saturation are observed and noted at baseline. The patient is asked to lift the tested arm and clench the fist, at which point the operator compresses both the ulnar and radial arteries, causing the disappearance of plethysmography waves. This maneuver allows the blood to drain from the hand. The hand subsequently is lowered, the fist is opened, and pressure over the ulnar artery is released. The Allen test is abnormal if ≥10 seconds are required for

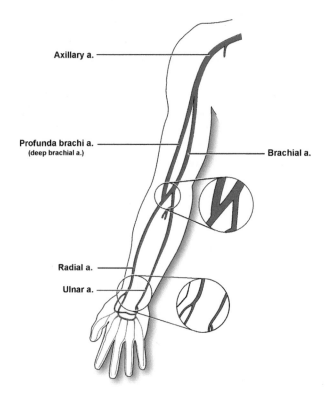

Axillary a.

Profunda brachi a.
(deep brachial a.)

Brachial a.

Radial a.

Ulnar a.

FIGURE 5.3   A diagram of the arm shows brachial and radial artery sites for needle access.

return of color to the hand. Plethysmography is observed for 2 minutes following release of the ulnar artery compression. The loss of pulse tracing with no recovery suggests an abnormal test and may suggest inappropriateness for radial catheterization, although this has become questionable after recent studies.[8,9]

After the site of access has been chosen, the patient's arm is abducted, and the wrist is hyperextended and fixed. The needle access site is prepared and draped under sterile conditions. The operator informs the patient that the procedure is starting. If the patient feels pain at any time during the procedure, he/she is instructed to notify the operator. The operator palpates the radial artery and identifies the point of maximal impulse, which is usually located 1 cm from the styloid process, where the artery is superficial and can be securely compressed if needed (Figure 5.3). Further tuning is done by placing the site of the maximal arterial impulse between the tips of the index and middle fingers. At this point, the operator keeps the tips of the fingers slightly spread apart, maintaining mild, steady pressure outlining the path of the radial artery.

The skin and superficial tissue over the access site are anesthetized with a 25-gauge needle containing 2–3 mL of 1% warm lidocaine solution. To cannulate the radial artery, the operator holds a 1.5-inch, 21-gauge needle lightly at the hub with the thumb and index fingers of the right hand (middle finger sometimes used to provide support for the needle), and inserts the needle at a 45-degree angle with the bevel pointed upwards through the skin at the site of maximal impulse between the left index and middle fingers.

The access needle is advanced until the initial pulsatile flow stops. Then the needle is slowly withdrawn to observe the return of pulsatile flow. Once the tip of the needle is in the arterial lumen, the J-tip, 0.02-inch, short guidewire is inserted and advanced through the needle into the vessel. The needle is then removed, and the 5-Fr Terumo pinnacle sheath on a dilator is advanced over the wire into the arterial lumen. To prevent arterial spasm, 3–5 mg of verapamil or 100–200 mcg nitroglycerine should be injected into the radial artery through the side port of the sheath. Heparin 40 units/kg bolus should be administered as soon as access is obtained in order to avoid sheath thrombosis.

Femoral Vein Approach

The right or left femoral vein is often used as access sites for diagnostic right heart catheterization (Figure 5.4) in the cardiac catheterization laboratory. The right femoral vein usually is chosen for general convenience. Identifying the position of the femoral vein in relation to the common femoral artery by vascular ultrasound prior to proceeding with cannulation is highly recommended.[10] After both of the patient's inguinal areas are appropriately prepared and draped under sterile conditions, the operator localizes the femoral arterial pulse as described above. The venous access site will be about 1.0–1.5 cm medial to and 1 cm inferior to the arterial pulsation. The skin and superficial tissue over the access site is anesthetized with a 25-gauge needle containing 5 mL of 1% warm lidocaine solution. After the tissue at the access site is well anesthetized, an 18-gauge needle connected to a 10 mL syringe with 2 mL of 1% lidocaine is inserted through the skin and is advanced at a 45- to 60-degree angle to the frontal plane with the tip pointing cephalad while a constant back pressure is maintained on the syringe. A single anterior venous wall stick should be the goal. Meanwhile, tips of the

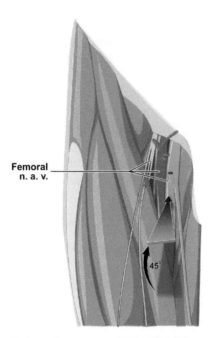

Femoral
n. a. v.

45°

FIGURE 5.4   A schematic shows the proper angle/direction of the access needle into the femoral vein.

operator's other hand's fingers maintain mild, steady pressure outlining the path of the common femoral artery. When venous blood flow into the syringe is observed, the syringe is tilted down to 30 degrees to the skin level and free aspiration of blood reconfirmed. The syringe is disconnected from the needle hub, and the operator ensures that blood return persists and is not pulsatile. The J-tip, 0.035-inch guidewire is inserted and advanced through the needle up into the vessel lumen. The needle is removed, and a small nick of the skin at the level of the guidewire entrance is made with a scalpel in order to ease the insertion of the 7- to 8-Fr sheath into the vein.

Once the sheath is appropriately positioned the dilator and the wire are removed, 2–3 mL venous blood is aspirated and the sheath is flushed with 10 mL normal saline.

Jugular Vein Approach

The right jugular vein is often used as the access sites for diagnostic right heart catheterization with or without endomyocardial biopsy.

The operator should spend time to position the patient correctly and comfortably in 15- to 30-degree Trendelenburg position, with the head rotated slightly to the left. After the patient's neck area is appropriately prepared and draped under sterile conditions, the operator informs the patient that the procedure is starting, and the patient will feel manual pressure, not pain, in the neck area.

There are 3 standard approaches to internal jugular vein cannulation; the most commonly used median approach will be discussed. Identifying the position of the jugular vein with vascular ultrasound prior to proceeding with any attempt of cannulation is highly recommended.[10]

MEDIAN APPROACH

The operator identifies as the anatomical landmarks the heads of the sternocleidomastoid muscle and the right clavicle (Figure 5.5). To better define the access site, the patient is asked to flex the head against resistance. The venous access site will be at the apex of the formed triangle. The right internal carotid artery can be palpated medial to this point.

The skin and superficial tissue over the access site is anesthetized with a 25-gauge needle containing 5 mL of 1% warm lidocaine

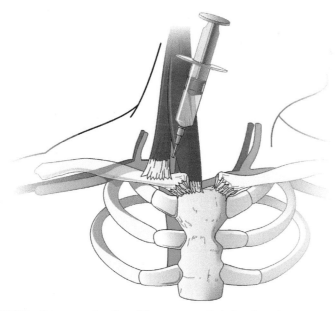

FIGURE 5.5   The proper direction of the access needle in jugular vein puncture are identified in the schematic.

solution. If the patient is slim, this is all that is needed to cover the anticipated access needle path. Otherwise, a 22-gauge "finder" needle and additional 5 mL of the anesthetic can be used to effectively numb the area in order to alleviate pain during the insertion of the 18-gauge needle. Care should be exercised to not inject the anesthetic into the vasculature. The "finder" needle, connected to a 5 mL syringe, should be employed initially to cannulate the vein. The needle should be inserted through the skin at the apex of the triangle and advanced at a 30- to 45-degree angle, with the frontal plane and the tip pointing towards the right hip of the patient while a constant back pressure is maintained on the syringe; venipuncture occurs within 2–4 cm. Further insertion of the needle should be avoided. When venous blood flow into the syringe is established, an 18-gauge introducer needle with an attached 5- to 10-mL syringe is inserted alongside the finder needle into the vein. The operator reconfirms the position of the tip of the 18-gauge needle by aspirating 2 mL of venous blood and asks the patient to exhale slowly and completely and then hold his breath. The syringe is disconnected from the needle hub, and the operator ensures that blood return persists and is not pulsatile. The J-tip guidewire is inserted and advanced through the needle into the vessel. Subsequent steps are similar to the femoral approach as described earlier.

Subclavian Vein Approach

The left or right subclavian veins are also used in the cardiac catheterization laboratory as access sites for diagnostic right heart catheterization. The operator should spend time to position the patient comfortably supine, in 15- to 30-degree Trendelenburg position with the head rotated slightly to the right and a rolled towel placed vertically between the scapulae. After the patient's right infraclavicular area is appropriately prepared and draped under sterile conditions, the operator informs the patient that the procedure has started, and the patient will feel manual pressure in the prepared area. An operator places the bevel of the venous access needle facing the numbers in the syringe in order to keep control of the bevel's position at all times. There are two standard approaches to the subclavian vein cannulation: supraclavicular and infraclavicular. The latter can be further subdivided into 3 variations: lateral, middle, and medial. The middle approach will be described.

THE INFRACLAVICULAR MIDDLE SEGMENT APPROACH

The operator identifies anatomical landmarks of the right clavicle and the suprasternal notch (Figure 5.6). The entire length of the clavicle is divided into 3 segments: proximal, mid, and lateral. The venous access site is 1–2 cm inferior to the midpoint of the clavicle. The skin and superficial tissue over the access site are anesthetized with a 25-gauge needle containing 5 mL of 1% warm lidocaine solution. To cover the anticipated access needle path, a 22-gauge needle and additional 5 mL of the anesthetic is needed to numb the area.

The 18-gauge needle should be inserted through the skin and advanced at a 10- to 15-degree angle to the skin with the tip pointing towards the clavicle and advanced until the bone is touched. Then the needle is withdrawn slightly and advanced under constant aspiration, just below the inferior border of the bone, in the direction of the suprasternal notch and parallel to the clavicle (Figure 5.6). When venous blood flow into the syringe is visualized, the operator asks the patient to exhale slowly and completely and then hold his/her breath. The syringe is disconnected from the needle hub. The operator ensures that there is no pulsatile blood return. The J-tip guidewire is inserted and advanced through the needle into the vessel. Subsequent steps are similar to the femoral approach as described earlier.

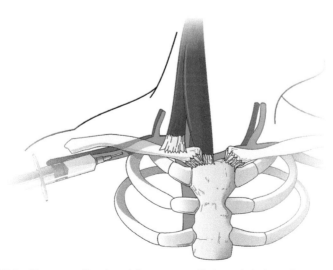

FIGURE 5.6   The proper direction of the access needle in a subclavian vein puncture are identified in the schematic.

Basilic Vein Approach

The right basilic vein can be used as an access site for diagnostic right heart catheterization. The skin is appropriately sterilized and superficial tissue over the access site is anesthetized with a 25-gauge needle containing 5 mL of 1% warm lidocaine solution. A micropuncture needle under ultrasound guidance is inserted into the medial branch of the brachial vein at a 30- to 45-degree angle (Figure 5.7). When the vein is punctured and venous blood backflow obtained, a floppy-tipped, 0.01-inch guidewire is inserted through the needle and advanced into the vein under fluoroscopic guidance. The wire should appear free and mobile to ensure that it is in the vessel lumen. When the 0.01-inch floppy-tipped wire is advanced into the basilic vein, the needle is removed. Next, a 4-Fr micropuncture sheath with a 3-Fr dilator is advanced over the wire into the basilic vein. The wire and dilator are then removed, and a regular, 0.03-inch guidewire is inserted into the micropuncture sheath and advanced through the basilic vein towards the axillary vein. The micropuncture sheath then is replaced with a standard 4- to 7-Fr sheath over the wire.

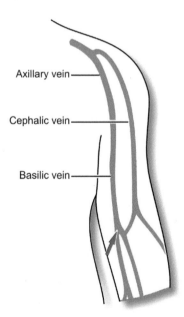

FIGURE 5.7   The proper access site in a basilic vein puncture is identified in the drawing.

WHAT IF AN OPERATOR ENCOUNTERS ONE OF THE FOLLOWING PROBLEMS?

Poor Arterial Blood Flow Return during the Arterial Needle Stick

Poor flow can be caused by severe peripheral vascular disease, low output states, or an incorrectly positioned needle tip. The proof for correct needle position is an unobstructed guidewire run through the vessel, or a "contrast-injection test" when a small amount of contrast is injected through the needle under fluoroscopy guidance to opacify the vessel lumen. Frequently when the operator is confronted with poor arterial blood return, the problem is in the position of the needle tip, which usually is located either subintimally, against the vessel wall, or in a small arterial branch. In such cases, advancing the guidewire through the needle tip will meet resistance, and the operator should not try to forcefully push the guidewire, rather reposition the needle after performing a contrast-injection test. If the needle tip has ended up in a small arterial branch, it should be removed and manual pressure held for 2–3 minutes until arterial hemostasis is achieved. If subintimal dissection is caused by the needle or by the guidewire, the site is abandoned, the patient observed for signs of an ischemic limb, and an alternative access site chosen (Figure 5.8).

J-Tip Guidewire Meets Resistance While Advanced Through the Access Needle

Occasionally, despite the brisk arterial blood backflow through the access needle, the guidewire fails to advance easily. This is a common problem when accessing a calcified, atherosclerotic artery. If brisk pulsatile flow is reconfirmed after withdrawal of the guidewire, the needle tip should be repositioned by changing the angle of entrance and its direction, or by slight advancement or withdrawal. A contrast-injection test can assist in repositioning of the needle. Usually, this problem is caused by the soft tip of the guidewire advancing around a sharp bend or a complex plaque. The needle should be withdrawn and manual compression of the access site applied for 2–3 minutes to achieve arterial hemostasis. The operator should not attempt to run a hydrophilic wire through the access needle, as inadvertent withdrawal of the wire may lead to vessel injury and possible loss of the wire into the vessel lumen.

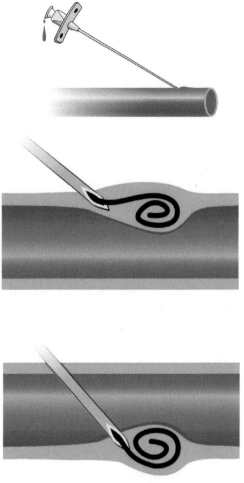

FIGURE 5.8 Anterior and posterior arterial wall subintimal dissection may occur either above or below the vessel lumen.

J-Tip Guidewire Meets Resistance While Moving Through a Deployed Sheath

Even after successfully obtaining arterial access and placing the sheath, there may be a problem of advancing the guidewire within the sheath. The most likely cause is sheath kinking (Figure 5.9A). The operator should slightly withdraw the sheath and rewire. If successful, the guidewire is followed by the catheter, and when it is placed safely in the vessel lumen, the sheath is advanced to the original position over the catheter. Alternatively, the sheath can be replaced with a kink-resistant sheath over the wire. If the wire still

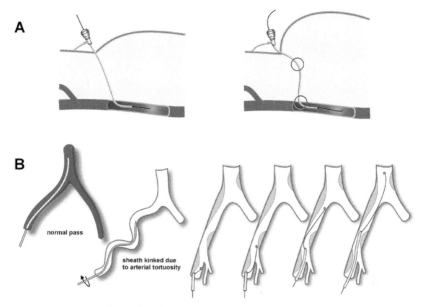

FIGURE 5.9   In Panels A and B, challenges in gaining arterial access are shown.

meets resistance within the sheath, the operator should recheck blood return. In case blood flows back, the next step is to flush the sheath and inject contrast dye under fluoroscopy to visualize the problem and make a decision based on the findings. If a kink cannot be straightened and a standard guidewire is unable to cross it, downsizing the wire can be attempted. If downsizing does not work, a catheter is placed over the wire and advanced as far as possible into the loop. When this occurs, the catheter and the wire are slightly withdrawn, facilitating the straightening of the kink. This method is especially helpful when dealing with a kink in a long sheath.

If blood cannot be aspirated, the problem may be related to loss of access. The sheath must be withdrawn and pressure applied. These problems can be solved by slight withdrawal of the sheath. The other cause can be clot formation at the tip or within the body of the catheter. In such cases, an attempt to save the access site can be made by putting the tip of the dilator through the membrane valve of the sheath and applying suction to aspirate the clot formed in the sheath. Every effort should be made to avoid moving the dilator distal to the sheath tip, because this can potentially dissect the vessel wall or cause clot migration into the vessel. If access cannot be saved after all efforts, the sheath should be removed and local pressure applied to obtain hemostasis.

J-Tip Guidewire Meets Resistance While Advancing Through the Blood Vessel

In cases when the common femoral artery is used as an access site, the problem is generally related to the tortuosity of the ileo-femoral vessel and/or the presence of severe atherosclerosis (Figure 5.9B). This can be documented on fluoroscopy by observing the path of the guidewire. In such cases, a sheath should be deployed as long as the guidewire is advanced for a few centimeters into the vessel lumen, allowing at least partial deployment of the sheath. After the sheath is deployed, blood is aspirated, the sheath flushed, and the sheath is then connected through its side port to the manifold. If the wire cannot be advanced, a small amount of contrast can be injected through the sheath and an angiogram taken in order to visualize the problem. In case of total obstruction, the sheath is removed, the site is abandoned, and manual pressure should be applied for 5 minutes until arterial hemostasis is achieved. On the other hand, if the obstruction is incomplete and can be crossed with the wire, an attempt to cross the lesion should be made. For the hydrophilic wire to run through the sheath, a 3-way stopcock is placed over the distal end of the wire and locked. This will allow easy maneuvering of a slippery wire using a swirling movement of the stopcock while moving the guidewire forward. When the stenosis is crossed by the guidewire, and if there is enough support to move the catheter over the wire, the stopcock is unlocked and removed from the guidewire tail. Then a 4-Fr Judkins right catheter is placed and advanced over the wire. If the sheath is only partially deployed, it is moved subsequently over the catheter into the blood vessel. In cases where the obstruction is located higher in the iliac artery, the Judkins Right (JR) catheter tip is brought close to the obstruction site. The guidewire is withdrawn and 1–2 mL of blood is aspirated from the catheter hub, which is then connected to the manifold. The catheter is flushed, pressure is recorded, and 5–8 mL contrast dye is injected to visualize the anatomy. If the obstruction is complete, the catheter and sheath are removed, the site is abandoned, and manual pressure is applied for arterial hemostasis.

If the obstruction is not complete, an attempt is made to cross this segment. Sometimes tortuosity of the iliac blood vessels creates problems for maneuvering of diagnostic catheters, and in such cases, a long, 45-cm, kink-resistant sheath is deployed in order to straighten the blood vessel. Occasionally, it may be challenging to deploy this long sheath in severely tortuous vessels without the support of a stiff guidewire. In such cases, the JR catheter is placed over the wire through the partially deployed long sheath. When the catheter is advanced sufficiently into the vessel, then the long sheath is deployed fully over the catheter.

In case of radial access, tortuosity extending from the radial artery all the way to the subclavian artery ("anaconda loop") can be an issue. After appropriate angiographic views have been taken to outline the brachial vessel loop, several different techniques can be used to address it. At first, the operator can try to downsize the wire to a 0.01-inch PTCA wire, or use a Terumo glidewire to cross the loop. If attempts to cross the loop fail, the site should be abandoned. Otherwise, after the catheter crosses the loop, the long 0.03-inch or 0.038-inch exchange guidewires should be used through the rest of the procedure. The major disadvantage of the smaller-diameter guidewires is their inability to provide enough support for the catheters to cross the loop over the wire. To deal with this problem "the buddy-wire technique" can be used by putting 1 or 2 additional 0.014-inch guidewires across the loop and then attempting to advance the catheter over these wires. If unsuccessful, one may attempt the "straighten the loop technique," where the catheter is placed over the wire and advanced as far as possible into the loop. Once this occurs, the catheter and wire are pulled back slightly, in some cases causing the straightening of the loop so that the catheter can be advanced. If this method fails, the "exchange the wire technique" can be utilized. For this method, after the loop has been crossed by the 0.014-inch PTCA guidewire, the catheter is advanced gently into the loop as far as possible, and the small-diameter guidewire is exchanged for a larger-diameter one. It is usually easier to negotiate the loop with a higher-diameter guidewire when the catheter tip is partially inside the loop. The other challenge for the operator is a significant tortuosity in the subclavian circulation or the presence of arteria lusoria (Figure 5.10).

In such cases it is very difficult to preserve the normal torque of the catheter so that the operator's eye-hand coordination and knowledge of different guidewires and catheters with unusual curves becomes important. In the presence of a tortuous subclavian artery, rotation of the catheter counterclockwise while the patient is taking a deep breath and turning the tip towards the ascending aorta in left anterior oblique (LAO) 45-degree projection facilitates access to the ascending aorta.

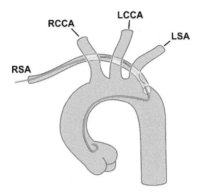

Arteria Lusoria

FIGURE 5.10 The presence of arteria lusoria creates a challenging procedure.

Sheath Meets Resistance While Advancing over the Guidewire into the Blood Vessel

The most obvious cause for this problem is an insufficient skin cut at the access site. A simple solution is to make a bigger nick of the skin before attempting to advance the sheath over the wire. The operator should avoid aggressive penetration with the scalpel to avoid lacerating the artery. The other obvious reason is placing the nick away from the point of needle entrance. The sheath is pulled back slightly, an appropriate skin nick is made, and the sheath is advanced over the guidewire.

In case of fibrosis of the vessel wall secondary to previous procedures, the operator withdraws the sheath and runs a dilator from the original sheath over the wire, then withdraws it and advances the original sheath with dilator over the wire into the vessel lumen. If resistance is still noted, the operator exchanges the regular sheath to a Terumo Pinnacle Sheath, with a smooth transition from the dilator to sheath, which usually solves the problem. If this sheath is not available, then the stiffer sheath can be attempted, which provides better support when advancing it over the wire. If all attempts to place the sheath fail, the operator may proceed with sheathless catheterization with the multipurpose catheter (see Chapter 7), or use the "telescopic" approach of a sheath (without dilator) placed over the catheter with the catheter diameter the same as the original sheath.

Occasionally, every attempt to place the sheath causes the guidewire to buckle at the arterial entrance. In such cases, the dilator can be placed over the wire into the artery, then the initial guidewire exchanged to a stiffer (e.g., 0.038-inch) one, and the sheath placed over the stiff wire with sufficient support. If a catheter or a dilator cannot be advanced over the wire, an attempt to perform a procedure from this site is abandoned.

If an artificial (Dacron) vessel graft was placed less than 3 months prior to cardiac catheterization, it should not be used as a site of access. Using a Terumo Pinnacle Sheath is highly recommended when accessing artificial grafts. If this sheath is not available, the access site can be predilated by using the dilator upsized by 1 Fr as compared to the sheath size planned to be deployed.

Bleeding Around the Sheath

The most frequent cause of this problem is a calcified blood vessel creating a "crack" at the site of sheath insertion. Another possibility is the laceration of the vessel with the tip of the access needle. The usual approach to this problem is to upgrade the existing sheath over the wire to the next-larger-diameter sheath.

Accidental Venous or Local Nerve Needle Stick

Accidental stick to either the median or femoral nerve causes sharp pain down the extremity. The most obvious causes for this are incorrect choice of the needle entry site or the wrong direction of its tip as it gets advanced. The needle should be withdrawn, and the point of access and/or direction of the needle tip advancement (in brachial, laterally; and for femoral, slightly medially) should be modified. If the operator accidentally enters the vein during the attempt to obtain femoral arterial access (unless the original plan was to perform right and left cardiac catheterization), the needle should be withdrawn, flushed, and after 1 minute of pressure hold for venous hemostasis, a second attempt to obtain arterial access made by aiming more laterally from the initial stick.

Radial Artery Spasm and Occlusion

Radial artery spasm usually manifests itself with severe forearm pain and new difficulty of manipulating the catheter and the arterial sheath. Occurrence of spasm has been reduced with appropriate use of hydrophilic-coated sheaths and the intra-arterial injection of a cocktail of vasodilators. If the patient keeps complaining of forearm pain despite the above precautions, a small amount of contrast after pressure check is administered in order to rule out vascular anomalies such as radio-ulnar loops or other anatomic variations of the upper-limb arteries. In general, adequate negotiation of radial tortuosity requires the use of a 0.014-inch hydrophilic wire, whereas tortuosity of larger caliber vessels can be negotiated by using 0.035-inch hydrophilic glidewires. Radial artery occlusion is manifested as asymptomatic loss of radial pulse and is generally prevented by using full anticoagulation with heparin and control of ACT. Immediate sheath removal after the completion of the procedure and a lower duration and intensity of radial artery compression during hemostasis decrease the chance of radial artery occlusion.

Accidental Arterial Puncture or Local Nerve Needle Stick

Accidental stick to a nerve causes sharp pain down the upper extremity. This type of complication occurs rarely with femoral access due to the lateral position of the nerve in relation to the vein. In rare cases, the femoral vein runs next to the artery or under the artery, which can be documented by vascular ultrasound. Rarely, the superior cervical ganglion can be damaged when attempting to perform internal jugular vein puncture, which could lead to Horner's syndrome (ipsilateral ptosis, miosis, and anhidrosis). There is no specific treatment for this syndrome. In some cases, permanent neurologic damage persists. If the operator accidentally enters the carotid artery during the attempt to obtain the internal jugular vein access, the needle should be withdrawn, and 2–3 minutes of manual pressure applied to secure arterial hemostasis. In patients with profound hypotension and/or significant arterial desaturation, it becomes harder to identify the pulsatile arterial flow, so an 18-gauge, single-lumen catheter should be inserted over the wire into the blood vessel lumen, which will not require a dilator. This catheter can then be connected to a pressure transducer to confirm the presence of venous waveforms and pressure. The most dreadful complication is accidentally placing the sheath over the wire in a noncompressible vessel like the subclavian artery. If this occurs, an angiographic picture of the artery should be obtained, and the sheath should be flushed and connected to the manifold for pressure monitoring. Certain closure devices can be used in most of the cases and vascular surgery should be consulted.

Pneumothorax

Incidents of pneumothorax can be managed by 100% O_2 therapy when small (<10%) and a follow-up chest x-ray done in 24 hours to ensure absence of progression. Otherwise, chest tube placement is indicated.

Air Embolism

To prevent this complication, catheter hubs should be closed at all times, and the patient should be placed in Trendelenburg position during sheath insertion if subclavian or internal jugular veins are chosen as access sites. If air embolism occurs, the patient should be placed in Trendelenburg position with left lateral decubitus tilt to prevent the movement of air into the right ventricular outflow tract, and 100% O_2 should be administered to accelerate the resorption of air. If the catheter is located in the heart, aspiration of air should be attempted.

References

1. Byrne RA, Cassese S, Linhardt M, Kastrati A. Vascular access and closure in coronary angiography and percutaneous intervention. *Nat Rev Cardiol.* 2013;10(1):27-40.

2. Kotowycz MA, Dzavik V. Radial artery patency after transradial catheterization. *Circ Cardovasc Interv.* 2012;5:127-133.

3. Sheth RA, Walker TG, Saad WE, et al. Quality improvement guidelines for vascular access and closure device use. *J Vasc Interv Radiol.* 2014;25(1):73-84.

4. Rao SV, Turi ZG, Wong SC, Brener SJ, Stone GW. Radial versus femoral access. *J Am Coll Cardiol.* 2013;62(17 Suppl):S11-20.

5. Casserly IP, Messenger JC. Technique and catheters. *Cardiol Clin.* 2009;27:417-432.

6. Criado FJ. Percutaneous arterial puncture and endoluminal access techniques for peripheral intervention. *J Inv Cardiol.* 1999;11(7):450-456.

7. Grollman JH, Marcus R. Transbrachial arteriography: techniques and complications. *Cardiovasc Intervent Radiol.* 1988;11:32-35.

8. Valgimigli M, Campo G, Penzo C, Tebaldi M, Biscaglia S, Ferrari R. Transradial coronary catheterization and intervention across the whole spectrum of Allen test results. *J Am Coll Cardiol.* 2014;63(18):1833-1841.

9. Bertrand OF, Carey PC, Gilchrist IC. Allen or no Allen: that is the question! *J Am Coll Cardiol.* 2014;63(18):1842-1844.

10. Weiner MM, Geldard P, Mittnacht AJ. Ultrasound-guided vascular access: a comprehensive review. *J Cardiothorac Vasc Anesth.* 2013;27(2):345-360.

Coronary, Renal, and Mesenteric Angiography

"Follow the rules, but avoid turning those rules into dogmas."

—Anonymous

Angiographic Views and Projections

Selective coronary angiography provides two-dimensional (2D) images of the three-dimensional (3D) coronary circulation. In order to better assess the presence and severity of coronary atherosclerosis in any particular segment of the coronary tree, the angiographer should use multiple angiographic views.[1-3] In general, there are certain standard views that provide optimal visualization of the particular coronary segment (Figure 6.1). Every angiographer should keep in mind that with each individual patient, he or she may need to slightly modify these standard views in order to obtain the optimal angiographic image.

Indications and Contraindications of the Procedures

The general indications and contraindications for left heart catheterization are listed in Tables 6.1 and 6.2.

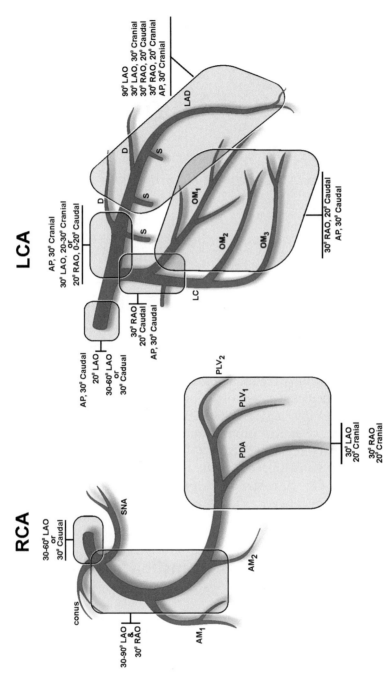

FIGURE 6.1   These standard angiographic views are used to visualize different segments of the coronary circulation.

TABLE 6.1 Indications for left heart catheterization and coronary and peripheral angiography.

Acute myocardial infarction	Particularly in individuals who will undergo PCI, are in cardiogenic shock, or have hemodynamic instability or mechanical complications and will need surgery. Persistent pain or unresolved ECG changes after thrombolytic therapy.
	1. In NSTEMI patients, if:
	   • Elevated troponin
	   • New ST depressions
	   • Heart failure
	   • Depressed LVEF
	   • Hemodynamic instability
	   • Sustained VT
	   • Previous CABG surgery
	2. Previous PCI in past 6 months

Unstable angina	Refractory to medical therapy
Chronic stable angina	Refractory to medical therapy or intolerant of antianginal therapy
Abnormal stress test	With high-risk criteria, even if asymptomatic • Positive at low work load < 6.5 METS • ST depressions ≥ 2 mm • Drop in BP > 10 mm Hg with exercise • Development of ventricular tachycardia (VT)/ventricular fibrillation (VF) • Transient ischemic dilation on nuclear imaging • LVEF drop > 10% • Multiple areas of ischemia
Ventricular tachycardia	Sustained
Left ventricular dysfunction	LVEF ≤ 40% of unknown cause
Valvular heart disease	Provide confirmatory data to Echo to assess outflow tract obstruction and quantify aortic and mitral regurgitation, and rule out CAD in preoperative work-up.
Preoperative assessment	Based on ACC/AHA/ESC guidelines. Also, before ascending aortic aneurysm or dissection surgery, as well as in patients with congenital heart disease, to assess shunts or to rule out coronary anomalies.
Hypertension	• Accompanied by "flush" pulmonary edema • In a young female patient • Newly developed severe and refractory • Noninvasive studies suggesting renal artery stenosis

Selective Cannulation of the Native Left Coronary Artery (LCA)

JUDKINS LEFT CORONARY CATHETER FOR FEMORAL, LEFT BRACHIAL, AND RADIAL APPROACHES

The Judkins Left (JL) catheter is a preformed catheter specifically designed to cannulate the ostium of the LCA without major

TABLE 6.2   Relative contraindications for left heart catheterization and coronary and peripheral angiography.*

Coagulopathy	For elective cases, INR < 1.8; heparin stopped 2 hours prior; platelets < 50,000 cells/mL
Renal failure	In dialysis patients, catheterization is generally scheduled after dialysis
Contrast allergy	
Infection	
Laboratory abnormalities	Anemia, hypokalemia, hyperkalemia
Decompensated heart failure	
Severe peripheral vascular disease	Synthetic vascular grafts younger than 6 months warrant special care; older vascular grafts increase risk of embolization of friable atheroma or thrombus
	Severe bleeding can occur if BP > 180/100 mm Hg

* All contraindications are relative contraindications.

manipulations. Clockwise and counterclockwise torque of the catheter will address an anterior and posterior orientation of the ostium of the left coronary artery (LCA) vessel, respectively. Superior or inferior position of the ostium should be managed through manipulation of the catheter in the vertical plane, or by changing the size of the catheter. In general, in patients with a normal-size aortic root, a JL4 catheter is used. In very tall patients (over 6 feet, 3 inches) or patients whose aortic root is known to be enlarged, JL5 or even JL6 may be tried from the start. Under fluoroscopic guidance, the operator advances the catheter over the J-tip guidewire through the arterial sheath to the aorta, keeping the tip of the wire protruding beyond the tip of the catheter in order to decrease the chance of aortic wall damage (retrograde dissection) and risk of distal embolization. Once the tip of the wire advances around the aortic arch, it is fixed above the sinotubular junction. The catheter slides over the wire until the tip of the wire is covered by the tip of the catheter, at which point the wire is withdrawn gently (to avoid abrupt "jump" of the catheter tip into the LCA ostium). A 5- to 10-mL syringe is attached to the proximal hub of the catheter, and 1–2 mL of blood is aspirated in order to clear the catheter from potential debris accumulation. If the operator has problems aspirating blood, gentle withdrawal of the catheter usually helps. The proximal end of the catheter is then attached to the manifold, and about 2 mL of blood is aspirated into the attached syringe, keeping the syringe at 45- to 60-degree angle elevation and simultaneously tapping gently on the manifold in order to remove potential air bubbles in the system. The catheter is flushed with normal saline, and aortic pressure is recorded.

Once pressure waves are recorded, the catheter is advanced under fluoroscopic guidance in a left anterior oblique (LAO) caudal view and with constant monitoring of aortic pressure. In the majority of patients, the tip of the catheter easily cannulates the ostium of the LCA; this can be noted on screen by a sudden "dive" of the catheter tip (Figure 6.2A). Occasionally, when the wire is being removed, the JL4 catheter folds into the aorta due to a very large aortic root and requires straightening and removal over the guidewire (Figure 6.2B). In the presence of normal pressure waveforms, the operator proceeds with 1–2 mL of contrast test injection under fluoroscopic guidance in LAO caudal projection. If the JL4 catheter ends up somewhat proximal to the ostium of the LCA, the operator can try the following approaches: First, a half-turn, clockwise rotation of the catheter with simultaneous slight advancement will work in cases where the tip of the catheter is not far from the ostium. However, if the tip is too far, the operator can either try to rewire the catheter all the way to the left coronary cusp (LCC) and, after removing the wire, attempt cannulating the ostium on slow catheter withdrawal. Alternatively, the catheter can be upsized to a JL5 or JL6. If the JL4 catheter tip ends distal to the ostium, counterclockwise rotation and slight withdrawal of the catheter often cannulates the ostium of the artery (Figure 6.2C). In other instances, the catheter should be downsized to a JL3.5 or even to a JL3.

In some cases, the ostium of the LCA has posterior, superior, or inferior orientation and is not engaged easily with a standard JL4 approach. Alternative catheters such as Amplatz Left (AL), JL3.5, or JL5 catheters may become handy. When the ostium of the LCA is intubated, pressure waves are observed to avoid "damping" (drop of amplitude of systolic pressure) (Figure 6.3A) or "ventricularization" (change in shape of aortic diastolic pressure form) (Figure 6.3B).

This is followed by efforts applied to place the tip of the catheter coaxial to the body of the left main (LM) trunk by advancing or withdrawing the catheter (Figure 6.4 A–B).

Once the catheter tip is placed coaxially with the LM trunk and the pressure tracing is appropriate, the operator sets the camera in right anterior oblique (RAO), 30-degree view with caudal 30-degree angulation view for the opening shot. The tip

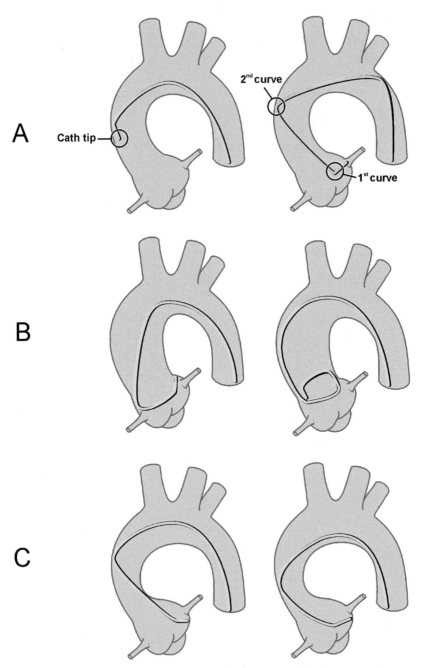

FIGURE 6.2 Schematic drawings show the steps and potential difficulties in engaging the LCA with a JL catheter. **Panel A**, a sudden "dive" of the catheter tip; **Panel B**, folding of the catheter into the aorta; **Panel C**, cannulation of the ostium of the artery after rotation and withdrawal (see text for details).

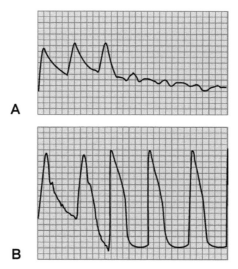

FIGURE 6.3   Hemodynamic patterns observed include "damping" (**Panel A**) and "ventricularization" (**Panel B**).

of the catheter on the fluoroscopic image screen is placed at a 10- to 11-o'clock position. The opening shot can be obtained using another view, if the operator chooses to do so based on clinical and previous angiographic data. The operator initiates cineangiography, turns off pressure, and injects 5–7 mL of contrast dye into the coronary artery under an initial slow rise, but using steady and constant pressure to opacify the coronary vessel lumen and to avoid streaming. Occasionally, prior to contrast injection a patient may be asked

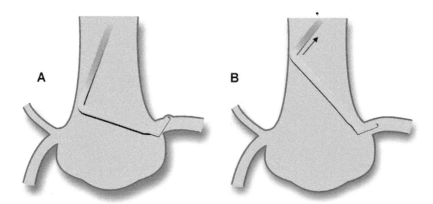

FIGURE 6.4   The potential problems illustrating the importance of coaxial positioning of the catheter tip in the LCA ostium are shown. In **Panel A**, incorrectly placed catheter against the vessel wall. Correct placement is shown in **Panel B**.

to hold his/her breath on maximal inspiration. This maneuver can reduce proximal vascular tortuosity and straighten the proximal vessel bends. When all of the appropriate images are obtained, the JL catheter is gently withdrawn below the aortic arch, the proximal end of the catheter is disconnected from the manifold, a 5- to 10-mL syringe is attached to the proximal hub of the catheter, and 1–2 mL of blood is aspirated. The operator advances the J-tip guidewire through the catheter under fluoroscopic guidance until the tip of the wire protrudes beyond the tip of the catheter, followed by simultaneous catheter and wire removal from the body through the arterial sheath. The arterial sheath is flushed with heparinized saline in the usual manner.

When utilizing the left brachial or radial approach, the operator may experience occasional difficulties placing the JL catheter due to the inability to navigate the J-tip guidewire into the ascending aorta. Certain maneuvers, such as turning the patient's head to the right, removing the pillow, extending the neck, abducting the left arm further from the body, performing the Valsalva maneuver, or just asking the patient to take a deep breath may facilitate guidewire placement and advancement of the catheter over the guidewire. If these maneuvers fail, a long, J-tip guidewire and the JR catheter can be used to navigate the wire towards the ascending aorta and subsequently exchange the JR for a JL catheter (Figure 6.5). This is technically accomplished in the following fashion: After the guidewire tip enters the aortic arch, it gets fixed, and the JR catheter runs over until it covers the tip of the guidewire. Then the operator, using the fingers of both hands, turns the catheter a half-turn clockwise until the tip of the catheter points towards the right shoulder of

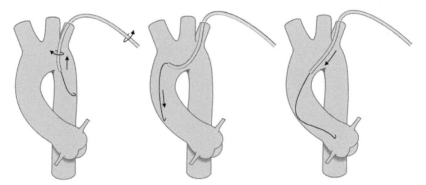

FIGURE 6.5 Operators can use the illustrated steps to overcome potential difficulties in engaging the ascending aorta from the left brachial or radial artery approach.

the patient. Next, the guidewire is advanced in the
the ascending aorta and down to the sinotubular jun
catheter is removed, and the JL catheter is advanced
towards the coronary cusps. The subsequent steps rep
have been described for the femoral approach.

With the right brachial or radial approach, the JL catheter is not
routinely used for engagement of the LCA ostium, as other catheters such as Amplatz Left (AL), Schoonmaker-King multipurpose,
Jacky (Terumo Medical Corp., Somerset, NJ), or Tiger catheters
have higher success rates. In those rare cases when the operator
still decides to proceed with a JL catheter, the J-tip guidewire is
navigated into the ascending aorta all the way down to the aortic
cusp, where the wire is forced to make a loop. The JL catheter is
advanced over the guidewire until its tip covers the guidewire tip.
Then the wire is removed, the catheter is gently pulled back and
clockwise torque is applied in order to cannulate the ostium of
the LCA.

Amplatz Coronary Catheter for Femoral, Left Brachial, or Radial Approaches

Amplatz catheters can be used to cannulate the ostia of the left and
right coronary arteries, but have a higher chance of causing ostial
injury in the hands of inexperienced operators. Although standard
coronary angiography can be done with these catheters, they are
routinely used in situations where the ostia of the left or right coronary arteries cannot be engaged with Judkins catheters due to
unusual take-offs (out of plane, high take-off, separate ostia, and
not originating from the appropriate coronary sinus).

LCA CANNULATION WITH AMPLATZ LEFT CATHETER VIA THE FEMORAL APPROACH

The choice of AL catheter size depends on the size of the aortic
root, with size 1 corresponding to a small aortic root, size 2 to the
regular aortic root, and size 3 to a large one. In order to cannulate
the LCA, the operator advances the catheter over the wire under
fluoroscopic guidance and positions its tip at the level of the sinotubular junction. Further steps for preparing the catheter are routine
and have been described earlier. Once these steps are completed,

the catheter (in LAO caudal projection) is advanced into the LCC without rotational manipulation of the tip. The secondary curve of the catheter ends up resting in the noncoronary cusp (NCC), while the primary curve and the tip are in the left cusp. Advancing the catheter with mild, counterclockwise torque forces the catheter to move up towards the LCA ostium (Figure 6.6).

Advancing and withdrawing the catheter moves the catheter tip in a vertical plane. It is important to remember that with catheter retraction, its tip has a tendency to damage the coronary ostium, so the operator should be aware of the pressure curve and catheter tip position at all times and, if in doubt, proceed with 1–2 mL of contrast test injection under fluoroscopy. As the tip of the catheter climbs up the wall of the coronary cusp, test injections in LAO and RAO projections can help the operator to establish the position of the left coronary ostium and its relation to the tip of the catheter. Based on this view, the operator makes a decision on the need to further advance or slightly rotate the catheter. When the tip of the catheter enters the LCA ostium, slight withdrawal of its body prevents displacement from the ostium. If the tip points up, the catheter should be pulled slightly back, and if the tip points down, the catheter is slightly advanced. The operator should avoid aggressively retracting or advancing the catheter tip into the LM trunk in order to avoid injury. Once the catheter tip is placed coaxially with the LM trunk and all appropriate angiographic images are obtained, the catheter is gently advanced, then clocked or counterclocked to disengage from the ostium in order to avoid dissection of the LM artery (Figure 6.7).

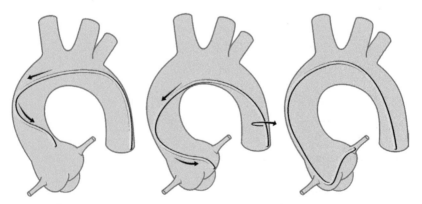

FIGURE 6.6   Operators can use the illustrated steps to cannulate the LCA using an AL catheter (see text for details).

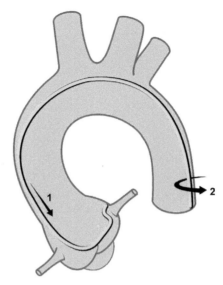

FIGURE 6.7   Operators can use the illustrated steps to properly disengage an AL catheter from the LCA ostium (see text for details).

LCA CANNULATION WITH AMPLATZ CATHETER VIA BRACHIAL OR RADIAL APPROACH

When utilizing the left brachial or radial approach, the operator may experience occasional difficulties placing the AL catheter due to the inability to navigate a J-tip guidewire into the ascending aorta. Maneuvers to overcome this problem have been described earlier. The subsequent steps repeat the femoral approach for AL catheter placement.

Selective Cannulation of the Native Right Coronary Artery (RCA)

JUDKINS RIGHT CORONARY CATHETER FOR FEMORAL, LEFT BRACHIAL, AND RADIAL APPROACHES

The cannulation of the ostium of the normally positioned right coronary artery (RCA) with a JR catheter requires manual dexterity. Two approaches will be described. When the ostium of the RCA is approached from above, the clockwise rotation of the catheter drops its tip down into the right coronary cusp (RCC), with frequent cannulation of the ostium of the artery. When the ostium of the RCA is approached from below, gentle pull back after clockwise rotation usually intubates the ostium of the artery. Despite these differences, the general technique for RCA cannulation with the JR catheter is very similar. The operator advances under fluoroscopic guidance the catheter over the J-tip guidewire through the arterial sheath to the aorta. Further steps for preparing the catheter have been described above. The JR catheter is advanced into the ascending aorta towards the RCC under fluoroscopic guidance in LAO 45-degree projection. In the RCC, the tip of the catheter should be facing the left shoulder of the patient. Under fluoroscopic guidance, the catheter is gently withdrawn approximately one intercostal space with simultaneous clockwise torque (Figure 6.8).

This slow, step-by-step, half-turn clockwise rotation should be done by the operator using the fingers of both hands, with the right hand on the catheter hub adaptor and the left hand assisting in turning the catheter near the end of the arterial sheath. After each turn, allow a short interval for transmission of the torque that is applied at the base of the catheter to its tip, just enough to point the catheter tip towards the right side of the patient's body. To facilitate this process, sometimes minimal in-and-out movement of the catheter is performed. This step-wise rotation allows the operator to avoid over-torqueing the catheter tip. The operator usually observes a small jump of the catheter tip when it cannulates the ostium of the

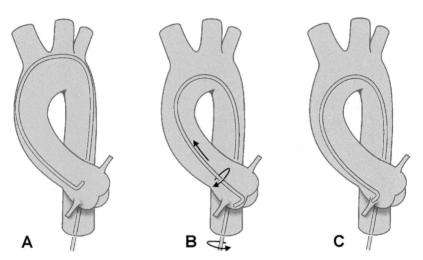

FIGURE 6.8   Operators can use the illustrated steps to cannulate the RCA using a JR catheter (see text for details).

coronary. In other cases, the operator notices a "catch" when the tip of the catheter gets fixed in the ostium of the artery. When RCA ostium cannulation is suspected, the pressure tracing is checked, and a small, half-turn, counterclockwise torque of the catheter is performed in order to neutralize the buildup of tension on the body of the catheter body by clockwise rotation. This movement will prevent the disengagement of the catheter tip from the coronary ostium. If the operator is not sure of the catheter tip position, test injections of 1–2 mL of contrast will assist in locating the ostium of the RCA. Occasionally, a separate origin of the conus branch, which is positioned anteriorly to the ostium of the RCA, complicates the clockwise approach. In such cases, counterclockwise rotation of the catheter with a posterior approach to the RCA ostium avoids cannulation of the conus branch and may help to solve the problem. In some cases, the ostium of the RCA is positioned high and anteriorly, or normally but with superior or inferior orientation and is not engaged easily with a standard JR4 catheter. In such cases, 3D-RCA, IMA, or right coronary bypass (RCB), MP and Amplatz catheters may become handy. When the RCA ostium is cannulated, pressure is checked, and further effort is applied in order to place the tip of the catheter coaxial to the proximal segment of the artery (Figure 6.9).

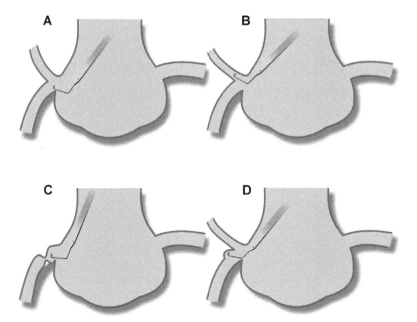

FIGURE 6.9 Drawings illustrate the importance of coaxial positioning of the catheter tip into the RCA ostium (see text for details).

Once this is done, the operator sets up the appropriate position for the tip of the catheter in the LAO 45-degree projection on the fluoroscopic image screen between 12 and 1 o'clock and initiates angiography. The operator then turns off pressure and injects 5–7 mL of contrast dye into the RCA. The opening shot can be obtained utilizing a different view based on clinical and previous angiographic data. When all the appropriate angiographic images are obtained, the JR catheter is gently withdrawn below the aortic arch. When utilizing a left brachial or radial approach, the steps repeat the femoral approach for the JR catheter.

RCA CANNULATION WITH A MODIFIED RIGHT AMPLATZ CATHETER VIA FEMORAL APPROACH

The technique of cannulation of the ostium of the normally positioned RCA with a modified Amplatz Right (AR) catheter is very similar to the one used for the JR catheter described earlier. After all appropriate angiographic images are obtained, the modified AR coronary catheter is gently pushed forward with clockwise rotation prior to disengagement of the RCA ostium.

When utilizing a left brachial or radial approach, the operator may experience occasional difficulties in navigating a J-tip guidewire into the ascending aorta. Maneuvers to overcome this problem are outlined earlier in the text. The subsequent steps repeat the femoral approach for a modified AR catheter.

RCA CANNULATION WITH THE LEFT AMPLATZ CATHETER

Although it is technically possible to cannulate the RCA with the AL catheter (Figure 6.10), these catheters are not used routinely for this purpose, and are mostly utilized when the RCA ostium has an anomalous origin in the aorta.

RIGHT BRACHIAL AND RADIAL ARTERY APPROACHES FOR SELECTIVE CORONARY ANGIOGRAPHY

When a right brachial or radial artery is used for selective coronary angiography, the technique of placing an AL or multipurpose catheter into the ostium of the LCA is not significantly different from the femoral approach described above.

One of the most frequently used catheters to cannulate both right and left coronary arteries from the right radial or brachial approach is the Tiger optitorque "Terumo" (Figure 3.10A).

1 **2** **3**

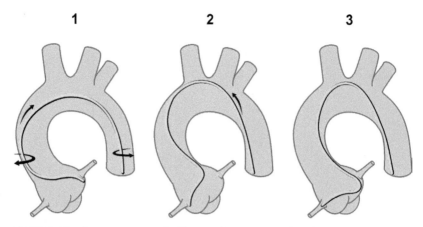

FIGURE 6.10   Operators can use the illustrated steps to cannulate the RCA using an AL catheter (see text for details).

As this catheter is placed in the LCC, it is flushed with normal saline and aortic pressure is monitored. The catheter is subsequently pulled back gently and torqued clockwise step-by-step with in-and-out motion to transmit the applied torque and to cannulate the ostium of the LCA (Figure 6.11A). After the artery has been cannulated and angiographic views obtained, the catheter is slowly withdrawn and disengaged. In order to cannulate the ostium of the RCA, the Tiger catheter is rotated clockwise and advanced to the RCC, where the operator continues step-by-step clockwise rotation of the catheter with simultaneous gentle pullback. This maneuver usually leads to successful RCA cannulation (Figure 6.11B).

There are different angiographic views utilized to obtain images of different segments of the coronary tree (Table 6.3; Figure 6.1). The decision of which angiographic view to use depends on clinical history and previous coronary angiography images, if available. In general, for the LCA, a RAO caudal view combined with LAO cranial view are chosen when biplane angiography is performed. These two views provide optimal visualization of the left anterior descending (LAD) artery and its septal and diagonal branches. For the RCA, plain LAO and RAO cranial views allow the operator to visualize the entire body, including the bifurcation segment and the right posterior descending artery (PDA). In order to improve the quality of coronary angiography when taking cranial views, the operator should ask the patient to take a deep breath and hold,

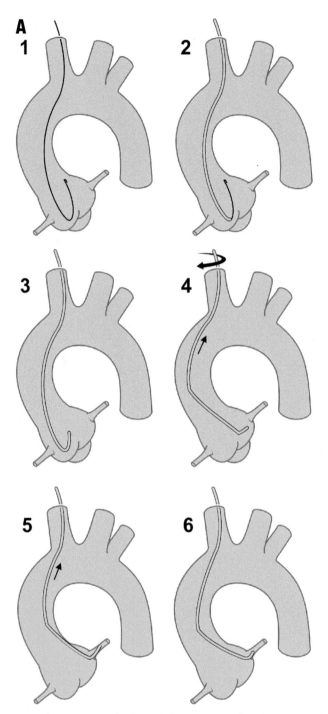

FIGURE 6.11   Operators can use the illustrated steps to cannulate the LCA (**Panel A**) and RCA (**Panel B**) using an Optitorque Tiger catheter (see text for details).

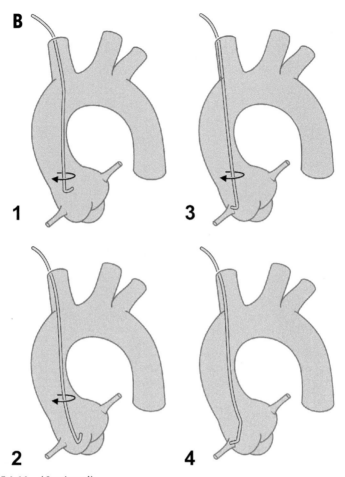

FIGURE 6.11 *(Continued)*

as this maneuver moves the diaphragm down and away from the angiographic field. The Valsalva maneuver should be avoided, since it pushes the diaphragm up.

Occasionally, additional angiographic views may be used to better visualize certain segments of the LCA (Table 6.4).

When obtaining different angiographic views the operator chooses appropriate magnification and corrects positioning of the screen in regards to the catheter tip in order to minimize aggressive panning (Table 6.5).

When obtaining cine images the operator should stay on the pedal long enough to be able to visualize all the late filling native vessels, coronary bypass grafts, and collateral circulation.

TABLE 6.3   Generally accepted angiographic views to visualize specific segments of the coronary tree.

PROJECTION / ANGLE	LCA
RAO 20°, caudal 20°	Left main, left circumflex, and obtuse marginal branches
RAO 30°, cranial 30°	LAD and septal perforators
PA, cranial 40°	Proximal/mid, mid, and distal LAD
LAO 45°, cranial 30°	LAD and diagonals
LAO 45°, caudal 30°	Left main, proximal LAD, proximal ramus intermedius, proximal left circumflex
LAO 90°	mid and distal LAD, septal perforators
PA, caudal 30°	Left main, left circumflex, obtuse marginals

PROJECTION / ANGLE	RCA
LAO 45°	ostium, proximal, and mid RCA
PA, cranial 40°	distal RCA, PDA, and PLV branches
RAO 30°	proximal/mid and mid RCA
LAO 90°	proximal/mid, mid, mid/distal RCA, conus, SA, and acute marginal branches
LAO 45°, caudal 30°	ostium, proximal, and mid RCA

TABLE 6.4   Additional angiographic views in LCA angiography.

PROJECTION / ANGLE	LCA
RAO 20° with minimal caudal 0–15° or cranial 20–30°	Distal left main and its bifurcation
LAO 20° with minimal cranial 0–15°	Ostium and proximal left main
LAO 45–60° with cranial 20–30° Over-rotated left lateral 100–110°	Ostial and proximal LAD Separates diagonal branches from LAD

Certain angiographic views can be used when specifically evaluating a particular collateral circulation (Figure 6.12; Table 6.6).

Selective Cannulation of the Renal and Mesenteric Arteries

The usual indication for selective angiography of the mesenteric arteries is clinical suspicion of mesenteric ischemia caused by a

TABLE 6.5 Correct positioning of the screen regarding the tip of the catheter in different angiographic views and the direction of panning.

PROJECTION / ANGLE	LCA POSITION OF THE CATHETER TIP AND DIRECTION OF PANNING
RAO 20°, caudal 20°	Tip of the catheter at 10–11 o'clock, pan table towards the operator and up
RAO 30°, cranial 30°	Tip of the catheter at 11 o'clock, pan table towards the operator and up
PA, cranial 40°	Tip of the catheter at 11 o'clock, pan table up
LAO 45°, cranial 30°	Tip of the catheter at 11–12 o'clock, pan table up
LAO 45°, caudal 30°	Tip of the catheter at the center of the screen, no panning
LAO 90°	Tip of the catheter at 12–1 o'clock, drop the table and pan up
PA, caudal 30°	Tip of the catheter at 9-10 o'clock, pan a table towards the operator and up

PROJECTION / ANGLE	RCA POSITION OF THE CATHETER TIP AND DIRECTION OF PANNING
LAO 45°	Tip of the catheter at 12–1 o'clock, pan table away from operator and up
PA, cranial 40°	Tip of the catheter at 12 o'clock, pan table towards the operator and up
RAO 30°	Tip of the catheter at 12 o'clock, pan table towards the operator and up
LAO 90°	Tip of the catheter at 12–1 o'clock, pan table up
LAO 45°, caudal 30°	Tip of the catheter at 12–1 o'clock, pan table towards the operator and slightly up

TABLE 6.6 Generally accepted angiographic views to visualize specific collaterals.

LCA INJECTION	COLLATERALS
RAO 20°, caudal 20° or RAO 30° or PA, caudal 30°	(left-to-right) LAD to PDA through septal perforators and/or through the distal tip collaterals (left-to-left) between septal perforators; between proximal LCX and distal LCX; between obtuse marginals; between ramus intermedius and obtuse marginals
LAO 45°, cranial 30°	(left-to-right) distal LCX to distal RCA; obtuse marginal to PLV branch; LAD to acute marginal (left-to-left) LAD to diagonals; LAD to obtuse marginals
RCA injection	Collaterals
LAO 45°, cranial 30°	(right-to-right) between conus artery and AV nodal artery (Kugel anastomosis); between acute marginal and PDA
RAO 30°	(right-to-right) between acute marginal branches; (right-to-left) between conus artery and proximal/mid LAD (so-called Vieussen ring); between acute marginal and distal LAD; between distal PDA and distal LAD; between PDA septal perforators and LAD septal perforators
LAO 45°, caudal 30°	(right-to-left) between distal RCA and distal LCX; between PLV and obtuse marginals

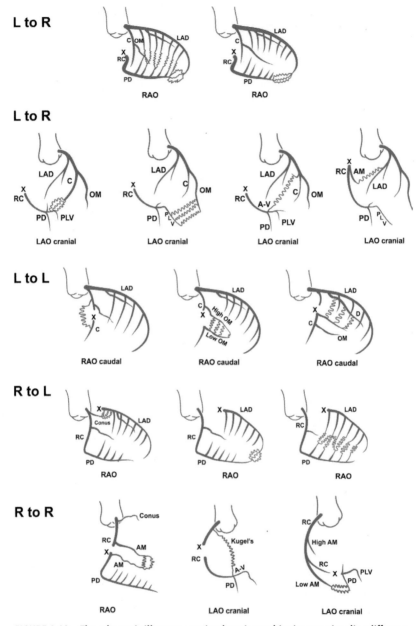

FIGURE 6.12 The schematic illustrates optimal angiographic views to visualize different collateral circulations.

AP

LAO

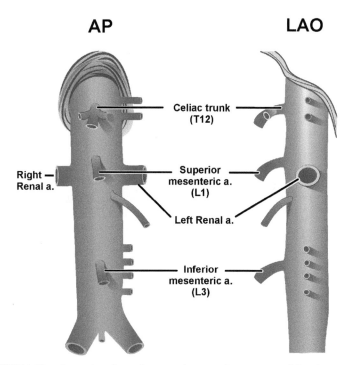

Celiac trunk
(T12)

Right Renal a.

Superior mesenteric a.
(L1)

Left Renal a.

Inferior mesenteric a.
(L3)

FIGURE 6.13   Illustration shows the AP and LAO 90-degree views of the abdominal aorta.

vascular problem (atherosclerosis, dissection, and thromboembolism). A major indication for selective renal angiography[4] is a work-up for severe hypertension suspected to be caused by renal artery stenosis or fibromuscular dysplasia. In general, if the contrast volume is not an issue, bi-plane (AP and LAO 90-degree views) abdominal aortography should be performed prior to selective cannulation of renal or mesenteric arteries. Due to the anatomic origin of the renal arteries, the AP view provides optimal visualization of these blood vessels. On the other hand, due to anterior aortic wall origins of the celiac trunk and the mesenteric arteries, the LAO 90-degree view will be the most suitable view for selective cannulation and evaluation of these blood vessels (Figure 6.13). This approach will allow the operator to evaluate the abdominal aorta and also provide a road map for further selective cannulation of the arteries of interest.

SELECTIVE CANNULATION OF THE RENAL ARTERIES

To cannulate selectively the right (slightly higher) and left renal arteries in PA view, the operator can use any of the following catheters: JR, IMA, RCB, and Cobra catheters. This view provides better visualization of the ostia of the renal arteries, originating from the abdominal aorta at the level of L1–L2 vertebrae. The J-tip guidewire is positioned at the level of T12 in PA view and fixed. The 4-Fr Cobra catheter (depicted Chapter 3, Figure 3.10C) slides over the guidewire, and the guidewire is removed. Test injection of contrast is performed under fluoroscopy in PA position to orient the operator to the position of the tip of the catheter and neighboring arteries. Then the operator slowly torques the catheter counterclockwise as one unit to point the catheter tip towards the right border of the aortic wall in PA projection (Figure 6.14A). To facilitate the transmission of torque to the tip of the catheter, minimal in-and-out movement of the catheter can be performed. The step-wise rotation allows the operator to avoid over-torqueing the catheter tip. As soon as the tip is appropriately positioned, the catheter is slowly pulled back until the tip of the catheter "snags" the

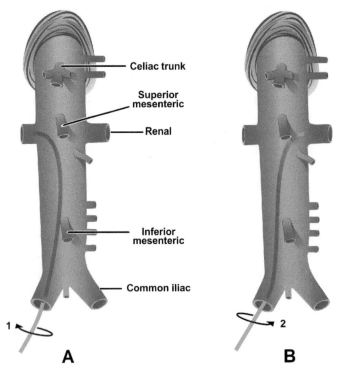

FIGURE 6.14   Selective cannulation of the left (**Panel A**) and right (**Panel B**) renal arteries is shown; the arrow shows direction of the catheter rotation (see text for details).

ostium of the right renal artery. Next, the operator makes a small, clockwise turn to eliminate the tension on the catheter created by the previous counterclockwise rotations. The operator checks the pressure tracing and, if normal, performs a test injection to assure the coaxial position of the tip of the catheter in the ostium of the right renal artery. Only after these precautions are taken is angiography performed in PA and contralateral oblique planes. After adequate views are obtained, turning the catheter clockwise takes the tip out of the right renal artery and points it toward the left side of the screen. Slight withdrawal of the catheter usually effectively cannulates the ostium of the left renal artery. The subsequent steps are identical to the previous maneuvers described above (Figure 6.14B).

SELECTIVE CANNULATION OF THE MESENTERIC ARTERIES

To cannulate the mesenteric arteries selectively, the operator usually uses a 4-Fr Cobra catheter and first cannulates the celiac trunk utilizing a left lateral view. This view provides better visualization of the ostium of the celiac trunk. The J-tip guidewire is positioned at the level of T11 in PA view, the 4-Fr Cobra catheter slides over, and the guidewire is removed. The catheter is flushed with normal saline, and the test injection is done under fluoroscopy in the left lateral position to orient the operator to the position of the tip of the catheter and neighboring arteries. The operator slowly turns the catheter step-by-step and counterclockwise as one unit under fluoroscopy, placing the catheter tip towards the anterior aortic wall on the screen. To facilitate the transmission of torque to the tip of the catheter, minimal in-and-out movement of the catheter is performed. As soon as the tip is appropriately positioned, the catheter is slowly withdrawn until the tip of the catheter "snags" the ostium of the celiac trunk (Figure 6.15A–B). Next, the operator makes a small, clockwise turn to eliminate the tension on the catheter created by the previous counterclockwise rotations. Then angiography in PA and LL projections are performed.

The approach to the superior and inferior mesenteric arteries is virtually identical to the approach described for the celiac trunk. The superior mesenteric artery originates just below the celiac artery, and is usually located at the level of the L1–L2 vertebrae. The inferior mesenteric artery sits even lower at the level of L3 vertebra. All of the mesenteric arteries originate from the anterior wall of the

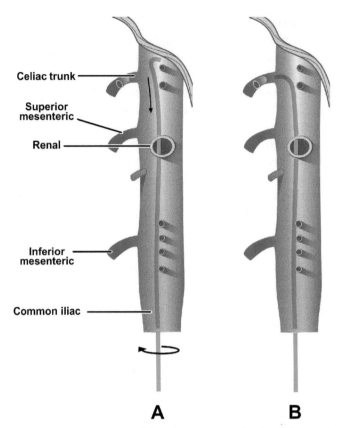

FIGURE 6.15 Selective cannulation of the celiac trunk: **Panel A** shows the initial advance of the catheter tip towards the anterior aortic wall, followed by withdrawal of the catheter to the point where it "snags" on the celiac trunk ostium. A small, clockwise turn brings it into correct position (**Panel B**) (see text for details).

abdominal aorta. Other catheters, including JR, IMA and RCB can also be used to cannulate the mesenteric arteries.

WHAT IF AN OPERATOR ENCOUNTERS ONE OF THE FOLLOWING PROBLEMS?

Arrhythmias

Prolonged episodes of arrhythmias in the cardiac catheterization laboratory are treated according to routine ACLS protocol. It is a widely accepted practice not to inject contrast vigorously into the conus artery or a small, nondominant RCA, or any coronary artery with tight ostial stenosis, since this can precipitate ventricular tachycardia and fibrillation. If sustained ventricular tachycardia develops while the defibrillator is being readied, the catheter can be placed in the left ventricle and "jiggled" a couple of times and the arrhythmia may stop.

A prolonged episode of bradycardia accompanied by hypotension, nausea, and sweating may be a manifestation of vasovagal reaction, especially in anxious patients with volume depletion. To treat this complication the operator should initiate rapid volume administration combined with intravenous 0.5–1.0 mg atropine and elevation of lower extremities. On rare occasions when hypotension is not responding to above measures, intravenous pressors can be used.

Pulmonary Edema

Pulmonary edema can be rarely a reaction to contrast injection,[5] but in the vast majority of cases, it follows the sudden increase in left ventricular end-diastolic pressure after contrast load in patients with more-than-mild systolic or diastolic dysfunction. Early signs are a ticklish sensation in the throat followed by dry cough and dyspnea, tachypnea, tachycardia, agitation, and the patient's attempt to sit up. The operator should intervene immediately and abort the development of this complication. Sublingual nitroglycerin, repeated as needed, accompanied with intravenous diuretics and oxygen through the facemask are effective measures. If not helpful, bilevel positive airway pressure (BiPAP) or endotracheal intubation with mechanical ventilation accompanied by intravenous vasodilators, diuretics and hemodynamic intra-aortic balloon pump (IABP) support may be required. Occasionally, as a desperate, quick measure, a large (60 mL) syringe can be attached to the manifold and 150–200 mL blood aspirated quickly.

Stroke

Stroke is a devastating complication of diagnostic cardiac catheterization.[6,7] The majority of strokes complicating diagnostic cardiac catheterization procedures are ischemic, and generally thought to occur as a result of embolism (blood clot, material from the atherosclerotic plaque, calcium from cardiac valves, air injected accidentally) or arterial dissection. The operator's vigilance during the procedure and postprocedural care helps to limit potential morbidity and mortality from periprocedural stroke. Early diagnosis and appropriate management involve neurology, neuroradiology, interventional neuroradiology, and, if needed, neurosurgery. If a stroke occurred during the procedure and was recognized by the operator performing the procedure, he/she first makes sure that airway, breathing, and circulation are stable, activates the stroke team, and makes sure that appropriate intravenous access is in place. Next, the operator sutures and secures the arterial sheath, orders emergency head noncontrast computed tomography to rule out hemorrhagic stroke, and performs a brief neurologic examination to localize the stroke, quantify deficits, and assist with choosing the appropriate therapy. If anticoagulation was given to a patient during diagnostic cardiac catheterization, it is not recommended to reverse it until after radiographic imaging of the head confirms a hemorrhage, since if the stroke is ischemic, acutely reversing anticoagulation can make the patient more prone to thrombosis. The decision on acute thrombolysis is based on the severity of stroke, presence of absolute contraindications to lytics, and time of recognition of symptoms of acute stroke (< 4.5 hours for intravenous thrombolysis with rt-PA, versus < 6 hours for selective intra-arterial rt-PA). In general, in the absence of absolute contraindications, if the clinical deficit is more than mild or not improving quickly, therapy with intravenous rt-PA should be initiated. Otherwise selective intra-arterial rt-PA or an endovascular mechanical approach with clot removal (time window up to 8 hours) can be performed by a neurointerventionalist.

Cortical Blindness

Cortical blindness is an extremely rare complication in contemporary diagnostic cardiac catheterization.[8] It has been described in selective vertebral or cerebral angiography both with high- and low-osmolar contrast, although it can occur with nonselective left subclavian or brachiocephalic trunk angiography. Cortical blindness occurs within the first 12 hours of angiography and is characterized by bilateral amblyopia or amaurosis with preservation of normal pupillary light reflex and extraocular movements. Accompanying clinical symptoms may vary and include headache, mental status changes, seizures, and memory loss. Computed tomography of the head reveals extravasation of contrast secondary to alteration of the blood-brain barrier due to increased permeability. The clinical course of cortical blindness is relatively benign, with complete recovery within several days without any specific therapy.

Myocardial Infarction

Myocardial infarction during diagnostic cardiac catheterization can occur but is relatively rare. It can be a result of embolism into the coronary tree, iatrogenic plaque rupture and thrombosis, or coronary dissection. Depending on the cause and severity, the initial approach may differ, but in most cases when a large artery is involved, the goal is to establish adequate flow via a percutaneous or surgical approach in a timely fashion.

Coronary, Renal, and Mesenteric Artery Dissection

Native coronary or bypass graft dissections are relatively rare with diagnostic cardiac catheterization, especially if small-diameter (4-Fr and 5-Fr) catheters are used. Patients with severe ostial disease when studied with large-diameter or aggressive-tip catheters (AL or AR) are predisposed to dissections. Vigorous contrast injection by the operator into a coronary artery where the catheter tip is not directed coaxially to the vessel wall is another cause of iatrogenic dissection. Careless manipulation of the 0.03-inch guidewire can also lead to dissection. Most acute dissections are ostial/proximal dissections with or without further propagation. Morphologically, dissections can be classified into 6 major groups (Table 6.7).

Left main coronary artery dissection can cause acute closure of the artery by the migrating intimal flap and can become one of the worst nightmares for a noninterventional invasive cardiologist. When left main dissection is recognized by the operator, immediate notification of the interventional cardiologist and cardiothoracic surgery team should follow. Simultaneously, an IABP should be set up for immediate placement, as well as a temporary transvenous pacemaker prepared for use. The only effective therapy

TABLE 6.7 National Heart, Lung, and Blood Institute (NHLBI) morphologic classification of coronary dissections.

CLASSIFICATION	DESCRIPTION
Type A	Minor radiolucent areas in the lumen without impairment of flow or persistent dye staining after contrast runoff
Type B	Luminal flap that is radiolucent and that runs parallel to the vessel wall with contrast injection but without impairment of flow or persistent dye staining after contrast runoff
Type C	Contrast appears outside of the vessel lumen as an "extraluminal cap"; staining appears even after contrast clears from the vessel
Type D	Spiral radiolucent luminal filling defects; often persistent staining after contrast clears from the vessel
Type E	New and persistent filling defects in the vessel lumen
Type F	Lesions that progress to impaired flow or total occlusion

for this complication is emergent CABG surgery or stenting of the left main artery. Iatrogenic spiral dissection of the native coronary or peripheral artery and bypass graft is another clinical situation which requires rapid stenting of the dissected segment of the vessel, and may prevent distal propagation and side branch occlusion with preservation of distal flow. Occasionally, ostial dissection of the native vessel or the venous graft may propagate into the ascending aorta and its management depends on the extent of the dissection. If the dissection involves the ipsilateral cusp and does not extend more than 4 cm into the aorta, it can be managed with stenting of the ostium of the involved vessel and close observation. On the other hand, any extension of the dissection more than 4 cm into the aorta requires surgical management.

Aortic Pressure Ventricularization or Damping

Aortic pressure that "ventricularizes" and or "damps" with cannulation of the artery is often encountered with end-hole coronary catheters. If the aortic pressure waveform shows the above mentioned changes after engagement of the LCA ostium, several potential causes should be considered, including selective engagement of the LAD or LCX artery, tight left main coronary artery stenosis, left main ostial spasm, catheter seated deeply inside the vessel, or the catheter placed against the wall. The latter 2 problems can be easily dealt with by slight withdrawal and, if needed, by fine rotation of the catheter tip for coaxial placement. Coronary vasospasm usually is treated by intracoronary injection of 200 mcg of nitroglycerin.

It is much harder and riskier to deal with severe left main stenosis. If suspected, the operator withdraws the catheter tip into the aorta and records the systolic gradient between the aortic and left main coronary artery pressure. The patient should be asked about symptoms and the ECG tracing examined. If the patient has no chest discomfort, vital signs are stable, and no ECG changes are observed, the invasive noninterventional cardiologist notifies cath lab personnel about the problem he/she faces, asking them to prepare the temporary transvenous pacemaker and IABP and makes sure that an interventional colleague is notified. Next, the operator may consider taking a nonselective cusp shot and, based on the obtained image, either exchange the JL catheter for another catheter with 1- or 2-Fr smaller diameter size and carefully re-engage the coronary ostium, or abstain from selective cannulation of the vessel, especially when adequate visualization of the coronary vessel and its distal branches has been obtained. If the decision is made to re-engage the ostium and no pressure and ECG changes occur with the re-engagement, and symptoms and vital signs of the patient remain stable, the operator can proceed with selective coronary angiography. On the other hand, if pressure changes, the operator may take one quick cine run with short injection of contrast utilizing a biplane camera set at RAO caudal or PA caudal combined with LAO cranial view with the goal of visualizing the distal vessel targets for potential CABG surgery. The catheter tip is withdrawn immediately into the aorta ("hit and run" technique). The operator should limit the number of engagements of the LCA ostium to avoid catastrophic consequences. An absence of contrast reflux back into the aorta during selective coronary angiography can be additional proof of severe left main stenosis.

Aortic Dissection

Aortic dissection is mostly retrograde and caused by aggressive manipulation of the catheter or guidewire. Most of such dissections are self-contained and self-healed and do not require surgical or percutaneous interventions.

Coronary or Peripheral Vessel Perforations

Vessel perforations are extremely rare with diagnostic catheterization and mostly seen in interventional practice. Management depends on severity of bleeding and use of antiplatelet and anticoagulant agents periprocedurally. Perfusion balloons, covered stents, and emergent surgery are potential treatment options.

Embolism

Air embolism in the vast majority of cases is due to the carelessness of the operator performing cardiac catheterization. Therefore, it can be prevented by meticulously following the general rules of angiography.[9] One particular point to emphasize is fluid-to-fluid connection of the manifold with the catheter. It is highly recommended with this technique to make sure that fluid flow from the manifold is very slow and "dribbling." This will prevent escaped air bubbles from traveling to the tip of the catheter while the operator connects the hub of the catheter to the manifold. If coronary arterial air embolism occurs, depending on the amount of air injected and symptoms of pain, electrical and hemodynamic instability may follow. In general, vigorous aspiration and flushing with saline and injection of intracoronary nitroglycerin are indicated.

Catheter Kinking, Knotting, and Clotting

Catheters of smaller diameter size (4-Fr and 5-Fr), with large curves, require more manipulation and are predisposed to kinking and rarely to knotting. The best remedy against such problems is prevention. While manipulating the catheter, an operator should carefully observe the signs of catheter knotting or kinking, such as sudden damping and flattening of the pressure curve and difficulty maneuvering the tip of the catheter despite applying clockwise or counterclockwise torque. When applying torque, the operator should help to transmit it to the tip of the catheter with small in-and-out movements of the catheter. If the operator suspects a problem at any time while maneuvering the catheter, the entire length of the catheter should be checked under fluoroscopy. Despite all preventive measures, catheter kinking/knotting can still occur. Most importantly, almost all kinks/knots can be untangled and removed intravascularly using specific devices, guidewires, and common sense. Thus, even if a complex knot or kink has been formed, the operator should approach it with a cool mind, patience, and with the understanding that the help of a vascular surgeon is rarely needed in such cases. Some of the following descriptions deal primarily with knotted angiographic arterial catheters.

To untie the large loop knot formed in the distal part of the catheter close to the tip, the operator attempts to anchor the tip of the catheter at the aortic wall while running the J-tip, 0.038-inch guidewire through the catheter carefully advancing the wire into the loop (Figure 6.16).

The key factor in the success of this procedure is simultaneous gentle advancement of the catheter while moving the guidewire through the knot. This may increase the size of the loop, gradually loosening and eventually untying the knot. The method frequently used to deal with small- or large-loop knotted angiography catheters is the "same-direction technique", which involves introduction of the untying catheter over the J-tip guidewire from a different access site but on the same side of the patient's body. The process of unknotting usually is done in the distal abdominal aorta, just above the bifurcation. When the tip of the untying catheter is positioned in close proximity to the small- or large-loop knot, the J-tip

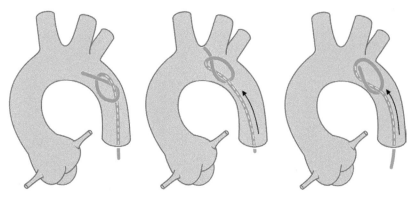

FIGURE 6.16   The drawing illustrates a technique for unwinding of a knot by catheter advancement (see text for details).

guidewire is followed by the untying JR4 or IMA catheter running through the knot by maneuvering the tip of the untying catheter. Next the operator runs an extra stiff wire through the knotted catheter all the way to the knot (Figure 6.17).

Then, the J-tip guidewire is exchanged to an extra stiff guidewire, which runs through the untying catheter providing extra support for this catheter. Gentle to-and-fro motion of the guidewire-supported knotted catheter against the guidewire-supported untying catheter may lead to gradual loosening and untying of the knot.

Simply pulling a knotted catheter through the vessel can cause severe vessel damage, so if the knot is too tight to untie, another means of removal is needed. If confronted with a tight, essentially no-loop knot in a 4-Fr angiographic catheter, the operator

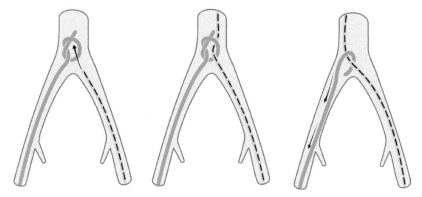

FIGURE 6.17   Another technique for unwinding a knot is by introducing another catheter (see text for details).

may attempt to make the knot even tighter, after which the initial introducer sheath is pulled all the way back over the catheter. The catheter is then moved back approximately another sheath length, and both sheath and catheter are cut at the hub of the sheath with sterile scissors. The original sheath is removed and a new sheath (2-Fr larger) is introduced over the catheter, maintaining constant control of the distal end of the catheter to prevent its migration into the vessel lumen. The idea is to pull the knotted catheter through the larger-diameter sheath, which is large enough to accommodate the knot. After the sheath is deployed, an attempt should be made to pull the knotted catheter through the sheath under fluoroscopy. If the knot does not fit well inside the sheath, the operator should not apply too much force, since this may lead to the formation of an "accordion" sheath, causing the sheath to collapse and subsequently damage the blood vessel. The operator should rather start by upgrading stepwise the sheath by 1-Fr and withdraw the knotted catheter into the sheath, with subsequent sheath removal. This approach works much better with venous access, and is primarily designed for this procedure. Occasionally, it can be used with arterial access if dealing with 4-Fr knotted catheters.

If the operator faces a complex kink, it should be moved into the descending or ideally into the distal abdominal aorta for judicious reverse rotation with or without stiff wire support and slow forward advancement of the wire as the catheter undergoes gradual untwisting. Some complex kinks require the introduction of additional devices such as a snare, vascular retrieval forceps, or a Dotter retriever inserted through the arterial sheath placed on the opposite side. The idea is to catch the distal tip of the kinked catheter and fix it with subsequent reverse rotation of the kinked catheter. This maneuver does not allow the tip of the catheter to continue spinning in the same direction as the base, which helps to untwist the catheter.

When catheter clotting is suspected, the operator should never attempt to flush the catheter. Instead, the catheter is moved back and rotated under fluoroscopy to prove that it is not placed against the vessel wall or inside a small branch. The next step is to check for presence of a kink anywhere along the catheter under fluoroscopy. If all the above steps are performed and the cause is not found, catheter clotting becomes a major concern. Any further maneuvers to open the clotted arterial catheter should be done in the external iliac artery to avoid embolization into the major cerebral, thoracic, or abdominal arteries. After pulling the catheter back to the lower external iliac artery, the operator cuts the catheter with sterile scissors at about 3–4 inches from the hub of the arterial sheath and observes the presence of spontaneous backflow through the catheter. If no flow is observed the clot is most likely located in the distal part of the catheter. In order to remove the clotted catheter, the operator may attempt to straighten the catheter using a thin, 0.018- to 0.021-inch guidewire, which is gently introduced through the catheter tip under fluoroscopy. There is always a risk of pushing an intra-catheter clot into the artery, but considering the small size of the wire, especially if working with 5-Fr or even 6-Fr catheters, the risk is small. The catheter is removed gently under fluoroscopy. In order to prevent clotting of the catheter or sheath it is very important to regularly aspirate and flush these tools with heparinized saline, not keeping guidewires in the artery more than 2 minutes, clean them regularly, and in cases where a prolonged procedure is anticipated or brachial access is utilized, systemically anticoagulate the patient with intravenous heparin bolus to keep ACT ≥ 200 seconds.

Poor Visualization of Proximal Segments of Coronary Arteries

Deep inspiration can reduce proximal vascular tortuosity, so asking patients to take a deep breath may help to straighten the proximal bend of the vessel and improve the quality of coronary angiography.

Other potential pitfalls and complications of the procedure can be found in Chapters 5 and 17.

References

1. Di Mario C, Sutaria N. Coronary angiography in the angioplasty era: projections with a meaning. *Heart.* 2005;91:968-976.

2. Patel MR, Bailey SR, Bonow RO, et al. ACCF/SCAI/AATS/AHA/ASE/ASNC/HFSA/HRS/SCCM/SCCT/SCMR/STS 2012 appropriate use criteria for diagnostic catheterization: a report of the American College of Cardiology Foundation Appropriate Use Criteria Task Force, Society for Cardiovascular Angiography and Interventions, American Association for Thoracic Surgery, American Heart Association, American Society of Echocardiography, American Society of Nuclear Cardiology, Heart Failure Society of America, Heart Rhythm Society, Society of Critical Care Medicine, Society of Cardiovascular Computed Tomography, Society for Cardiovascular Magnetic Resonance, and Society of Thoracic Surgeons. *J Am Coll Cardiol.* 2012;59(22):1995-2027.

3. Casserly IP, Messenger JC. Technique and catheters. *Cardiol Clin.* 2009;27:417-432.

4. White CJ, Jaff MR, Haskal ZJ, et al. Indications for renal arteriography at the time of coronary arteriography: a science advisory from the American Heart Association Committee on Diagnostic and Interventional Cardiac Catheterization, Council on Clinical Cardiology, and the Councils on Cardiovascular Radiology and Intervention and on Kidney in Cardiovascular Disease. *Circulation.* 2006;114:1892-1895.

5. Paul RE. Fatal non-cardiogenic pulmonary edema after intravenous non-ionic radiographic contrast. *Lancet.* 2002;359(9311):1037-1037.

6. Werner N, Zahn R, Zeymer U. Stroke in patients undergoing coronary angiography and percutaneous coronary intervention: incidence, predictors, outcome and therapeutic options. *Expert Rev Cardiovasc Ther.* 2012;10(10):1297-1305.

7. Hamon M, Baron JC, Viader F, Hamon M. Periprocedural stroke and catheterization. *Circulation.* 2008;118(678-683).

8. Math RS, Singh S, Bahl V. An uncommon complication after a common procedure. *J Invasive Cardiol.* 2008;20(10):E301-E303.

9. Dib J, Boyle AJ, Chan M, Resar JR. Coronary air embolism: a case report and review of the literature. *Cathet Cardiovasc Intervent.* 2006;68:897-900.

CHAPTER 7

The Multipurpose Catheter

"Practice is everything."

—Periander

Historical Background

The multipurpose catheter technique was introduced to Emory University Cardiac Catheterization Laboratories in 1972 by Spencer King. King learned this method from Fred Schoonmaker in Denver, Colorado.[1] At Emory, the technique was further learned and later taught by John Douglas. The technique has been described also in a book published by King and Douglas.[2] The descriptions of this method in this chapter attempt to add a few small points that have been picked up through the years by one of the authors (SDC) such that they can be passed on to individuals interested to learn this technique.[3]

It was the dream of Andreas Gruentzig that cardiac catheterization be performed as an outpatient with small catheters. He himself underwent a cardiac catheterization with small catheters performed by a cardiology fellow, Whit Whitworth, in order to prove that it could be done. After the procedure, he had a couple of hours of bed rest and went out dancing. That evening he developed a hematoma that caused him to hold pressure and take some more bed rest.

Gruentzig's dream was also to have a cardiac catheterization laboratory dedicated to low-risk outpatients who could go directly to cardiac catheterization as a first procedure. In the early 1980s, this concept was realized. The Fisher Company had promised to provide Gruentzig and Emory the equipment (which was all digital), and plans were made to create a laboratory. A location was chosen in the tunnel level of Building A of The Emory Clinic, and construction was initiated. Unfortunately, Gruentzig lost his life in a plane crash in 1985 and never saw the laboratory completed.

The laboratory was opened in 1986 with the principles of Gruentzig in mind, and in the beginning, 4-Fr and 5-Fr Judkins catheters were used. These catheters were small and posed difficulty when used in large patients, those with aortic valve disease, and those with aortic ectasia. They were simply blown away by aortic stenosis/regurgitation jets and large stroke volumes. The 6-Fr multipurpose catheter came to the forefront because of its maneuverability and slightly larger inner diameter and was used originally without a sheath. The multipurpose catheter had been developed by Schoonmaker in 7-Fr and 8-Fr sizes. It was not until the outpatient concept was proven possible that the 6-Fr multipurpose catheter became popular. This led to smaller guiding systems for intervention in the 6-Fr size.

Currently, the 5-Fr multipurpose catheter is available and can be used in straightforward situations. Manipulation can be difficult because it kinks easily, does not take torque and rotation well, and is easily blown away by the flow jets of aortic stenosis and regurgitation as mentioned above.

The 6-Fr multipurpose catheter has stood the test of time at Emory for outpatient cardiac catheterization. Experience with the first 3,000 patients was reported in 1991,[3] and to date more than 26,000 low-risk patients in the Andreas Gruentzig Outpatient Laboratory have been done with these catheters. With the increased use of closure devices, almost all patients are discharged home earlier and more comfortably after diagnostic cardiac catheterization.

Multipurpose Catheter Basics

Once femoral access has been obtained and a sheath is inserted, the J-tip guidewire should be advanced across the arch with the catheter following into the ascending aorta as discussed in previous chapters. The monitoring of catheter and wire placement into the ascending aorta should be done under fluoroscopic guidance in the RAO or LAO position. The wire should be removed, the catheter aspirated and connected to the manifold, and the catheter should be flushed. Care should be taken as the catheter–manifold connection is made to minimize any air entry in the system. The syringe should be checked for air by careful inspection and tapping upon it to move any bubbles toward the top of the syringe. It is safer to make the catheter–manifold connection with the heparinized saline port flowing forward in order to minimize any introduction of air. The syringe should have no bubbles to ensure a "bubble-free environment" and to prevent injection of microbubbles later. Once these connections are made, several aspirations and flushes should be made before the syringe is filled with contrast. Always watch for bubbles—even the contrast line can contain a few. When the contrast bottle is nearing empty and needs replacing, it is always good to replace the bottle before it is completely empty so as to avoid getting air within the system.

Torque and Rotation

The concepts of torque and rotation are important to understand as one learns the multipurpose technique. Both are necessary for success with this catheter. Torque is used to make rotation of the catheter tip happen. Torque may be applied to the catheter near the sheath edge by the left hand, but frequently rotation of the catheter tip will not occur until the catheter is moved slightly in and out of the sheath, transmitting the torque. The catheter is bound in several places, including the sheath, the iliac arteries, the aortic arch, and the point where the catheter touches the aortic wall. When torque is applied to the catheter, potential rotation builds up and will not release until the catheter is moved slightly in and out of the sheath. This effectively frees up the wire-braded catheter, allowing torque to be translated into rotation. Sometimes torque builds up so much that the catheter "helicopters" around in the ascending aorta, which is an undesirable event. The smaller the catheter, the more easily torque is stored, and the more spring-like it becomes. Larger catheters behave more like rods (i.e., rotation at the hub results in rotation at the tip). If torque is applied vigorously without tip rotation occurring, the catheter can kink and the arterial pressure will appear damped, or worse, a knot can form in the catheter (usually in the distal aorta or iliac arteries). This should be removed by reversing the direction of the initial torque until the kink is unwound (see also

Chapter 6 for more details). Appreciation of these principles aids in learning how to manipulate both large and small catheters.

The manner in which the multipurpose catheter and manifold are held and manipulated is different from the conventional Judkins technique as described in Chapter 6. All catheter manipulations, including advancement, withdrawal, and torque application and rotation, are usually made with the left hand from the hub or most proximal part of the catheter at the sheath. The injection syringe and manifold are held with the right hand (Figure 7.1).

This arrangement permits easy administration of small "tests" or puffs of contrast as the catheter position is changed with the pressure in the off position. When first learning this technique, it is best to use two hands on the catheter. The right hand is placed on the manifold with the thumb and index finger on the end of the manifold and hub of the catheter such that it can be rotated. The left hand is placed on the catheter close to the hub of the sheath. Rotation can be applied at the hub and then the left hand can transfer this rotation through the sheath and thus causing the tip of the catheter to move in the desirable location. The left hand can move the catheter in and out of the sheath to facilitate transfer of torque (Figure 7.2).

As part of the catheterization procedure, one should always be watchful of the pressure tracings looking for damping or significant elevations or decreases in blood pressure. Each time the coronary artery is engaged or the catheter is positioned within the left ventricle, the pressure should be checked watching for damping or ventricularization of the pressure waveform. If the pressure is not normal, the catheter is obstructing an artery or is entrapped within the left ventricle. A small puff of contrast can also be helpful. Rapid run-off means that the catheter is not obstructing the artery and a full injection can be made safely.

Left Ventriculography with the Multipurpose Catheter

From the RAO position, the catheter can be advanced into the left ventricle. Sometimes, from the right coronary cusp (RCC), the catheter can be moved up and down, and with slight counterclockwise torque, it will fall across the aortic valve into the left ventricle.

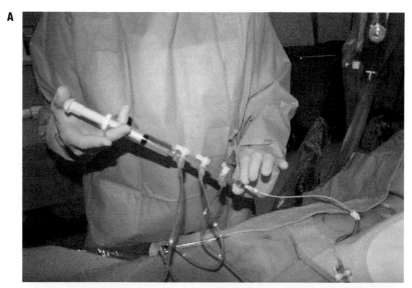

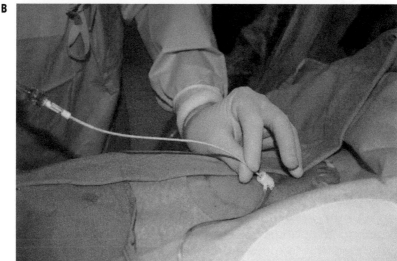

FIGURE 7.1   Shown are illustrations of how to hold and manipulate (**Panel A**) the hub of the multipurpose catheter and (**Panel B**) the multipurpose catheter at the sheath. **Panel A**: The hub of the catheter is rotated which applies torque to the shaft of the catheter. The torque in the shaft of the catheter can then be transferred to the tip of the catheter with the left hand at the sheath hub. **Panel B**: The left hand is grasping the catheter near the sheath and manipulating the catheter as needed to transfer the torque that was previously applied to the catheter at the hub to the tip of the catheter.

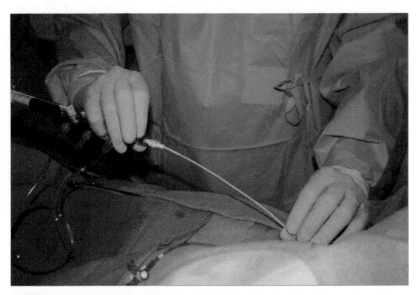

FIGURE 7.2   The two-handed method consists of the following: The right hand is applying torque at the hub as the left hand manipulates this further at the sheath, transferring the torque through the sheath to the tip of the catheter.

Otherwise, a loop can be made by counterclockwise rotation of the catheter so that it points posteriorly in the ascending aorta into the noncoronary cusp (NCC). Advancing with a small amount of clockwise torsion will then allow the catheter to form a loop and flip anterior, sometimes landing in the left coronary cusp (LCC). If the catheter fails to drop into the LCC, a loop will be formed above the sinotubular ridge. The catheter should then be rotated clockwise such that the tip points away from the operator (Figure 7.3).

From this position, the loop can usually be advanced across the aortic cusp area into the left ventricle. The "knee" of the catheter will usually fall between the commissures and allow the catheter to prolapse into the left ventricle. The RAO view is favored for crossing into the left ventricle in order to prevent the tip of the multipurpose catheter from pointing too anteriorly and inadvertently entering into and passing down the right coronary artery (RCA) when it is advanced. Once in the left ventricle, the tip of the catheter should point slightly upward or superior and there should be slight up and down mobility indicating that it is free from the wall (Figure 7.4).

In the LAO projection, the catheter should be directed slightly away from the septum. At this point, the left ventricular end-diastolic pressure (LVEDP) can be measured and ventriculography

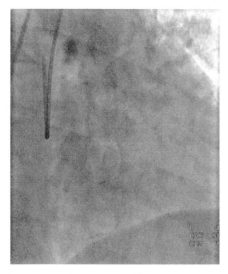

FIGURE 7.3   The multipurpose catheter is viewed from the RAO position. The loop is formed and points directly away from the operator poised to be prolapsed across the aortic valve or ready to drop down into the LCC when pulled up.

performed. It is always important to give a small test injection to ensure that the catheter tip is moving freely before ventriculography. A hand injection is usually adequate. For the best image, the patient should be asked to take about half a breath and "stop

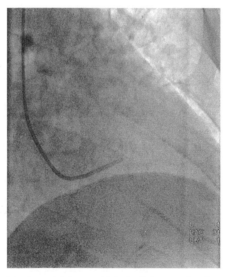

FIGURE 7.4   The multipurpose catheter within the left ventricle: The tip is pointing slightly anterior and moves freely. If the tip is not freely mobile, this indicates that the tip is stuck within either the chords or the trabeculations.

breathing" to keep the background still while the injection is done. If one asks the patient to "take a deep breath and hold it," they frequently take a breath and do a Valsalva maneuver, which alters the dynamics of the situation and elevates the diaphragm.

▶ Video 7.1 shows left ventriculography with the multipurpose catheter in RAO projection, and ▶ Video 7.2 shows left ventriculography with the multipurpose catheter in LAO projection. An incorrect position of the multipurpose catheter for left ventriculography is featured in ▶ Video 7.3.

If a power injection is required due to a large ventricular chamber or to more accurately assess mitral regurgitation, a pigtail catheter is favored. After ventriculography, the contrast is flushed from the catheter for an accurate post-ventriculography LVEDP. Then the catheter can be withdrawn back into the aorta with the pressure turned on, noting the presence or absence of a gradient.

Right Coronary Artery (RCA) Cannulation

The RCA is cannulated by placing the catheter tip in the RCC from the RAO view. Clockwise rotation will result in the catheter moving anterior and into the RCC.

▶ Video 7.4 shows engagement of the RCA ostium with the multipurpose catheter in RAO projection. Then the catheter should be further manipulated from the LAO view, where two approaches are possible. The first is to view the catheter from the LAO position and simply pull back and rotate the tip clockwise from a position just above the RCC, exactly as is done with a JR catheter (Figure 7.5A). The second approach is to advance the catheter in the RCC from the 6 o'clock position in the LAO view watching for it to flatten out and allowing the tip to move toward and into the ostium of the RCA.

Puffs of contrast can be used to better locate the position of the ostium (Figure 7.6). One should remember that the ostium of the RCA can be located in the bottom of the cusp, in the midportion of the cusp, at the sinotubular ridge, or it can arise in an unusual position as an anomaly.

▶ Video 7.5 shows engagement of the RCA with the multipurpose catheter in RAO projection. This can be done much like one does with the JR catheter as described in Chapter 6. It is easier to do

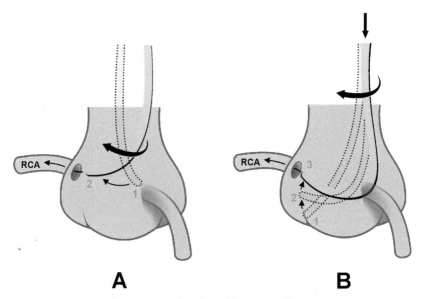

A **B**

FIGURE 7.5   To cannulate the RCA using the multipurpose catheter, an operator can either pull back and rotate the catheter tip from just above the RCC in LAO view **(Panel A)** or advance the catheter in the RCC from the 6 o'clock position in the LAO view watching for it to flatten out and allowing the tip to move toward and into the ostium of the RCA **(Panel B)**.

when the RCA has an inferior orientation from the ostium rather than a superior orientation as seen above.

▶ Video 7.6 shows cannulation of the RCA with the multipurpose catheter in LAO projection. This method of cannulation may be more easily done if the first segment of the RCA is inferiorly oriented. However, if the first segment is oriented in a superior direction, it is still possible. Even right coronary arteries with an anterior take-off can be engaged with the multipurpose catheter using this "sweep-around" technique (Figure 7.7). Sometimes, when this anatomy is present, one can be deep within the artery before one realizes. When the pressure damps with clockwise rotation of the catheter, this might be the situation.

In order to get the catheter tip to move around in the aorta, the catheter tip must be above the level of the aortic cusps. One can rotate the catheter in the NCC and never get the tip out of the sinus of Valsalva. Rotation without withdrawal will result in the catheter not leaving the NCC or diving down to a position below the ostium of the RCA. As one rotates, one has to withdraw in order to keep the tip at the same level in the ascending aorta or the sinuses.

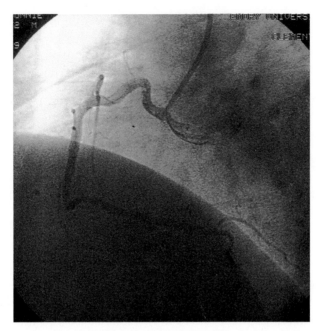

FIGURE 7.6   Cannulation of the RCA with the multipurpose catheter is performed by sweeping around and slightly withdrawing the catheter, allowing the tip to engage the RCA.

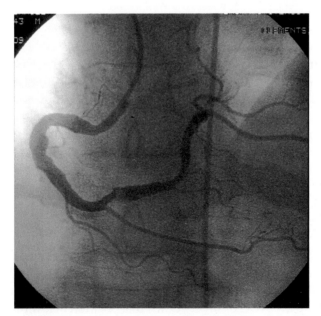

FIGURE 7.7   Engagement of the RCA with the multipurpose catheter is achieved by sweeping around from the LAO view. This RCA ostium has a more anterior location, a situation that is more difficult to cannulate with a JR catheter.

The second approach is to advance the catheter in the RCC from the 6-o'clock position (Figure 7.8) in the LAO view, watching for it to flatten out and allowing the tip to move toward and into the ostium of the RCA. If this second maneuver is unsuccessful from the 6-o'clock position, the catheter tip should be rotated to a position just below the ostium of the RCA and then advanced.

This maneuver should form a loop with the tip oriented toward the ostium of the RCA. As one manipulates the catheter (typically with the left hand), a small puff of contrast is helpful to identify the position of the tip relative to the ostium of the RCA. Details of this second approach are explained in the following paragraphs.

As one uses the second method of advancing in the cusp, starting at the 6-o'clock position is very important. The first step is to place the catheter in the RCC from the RAO view (Figure 7.9) and then moving to the LAO view. Invariably, the catheter will be short of the 6-o'clock position (Figure 7.10), and a slight amount of clockwise rotation is needed until the catheter points straight down at 6 o'clock in the LAO view (Figure 7.11). Once in the LAO view, gently rotate the catheter to this point. When this position is obtained, no torque should be on the catheter.

When using the second method of "advancing in the cusp," the catheter should be advanced with the left hand using small puffs

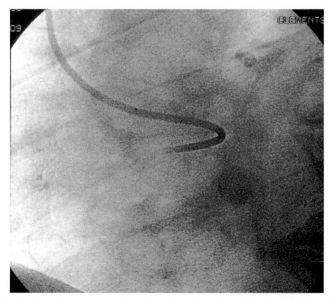

FIGURE 7.8   The multipurpose catheter is ready to be advanced to the ostium of the RCA. This position is obtained by advancing from the 6-o'clock position from the LAO view.

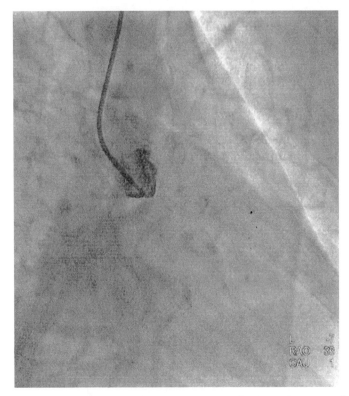

FIGURE 7.9   The image shows the multipurpose catheter after having been rotated clockwise to this anterior position and tested with a puff of contrast. This is indicating the correct orientation from this view. The next step is to go to the LAO view.

in the "off-pressure" mode, watching for the catheter tip to move toward the ostium of the RCA. Sometimes it will move gently in that direction, and other times it will "dart" over toward the ostium (Figure 7.5B). Once it contacts the ostium, the catheter can be stabilized by slight withdrawal. This may actually result in the catheter going further down into the ostium. If this occurs, more withdrawal is necessary until the catheter becomes stable. If the catheter tip lands high above the RCA ostium using the second approach, it should be withdrawn slightly and a small amount of clockwise torque applied to the catheter at the sheath, which is transferred to the tip by simple advancement. This should result in a more inferior position, frequently landing in the ostium of the RCA. If the catheter tip lands in a low position relative to the ostium of the RCA, slight withdrawal of the catheter at the sheath with the left hand and application of a small amount of counterclockwise torque will

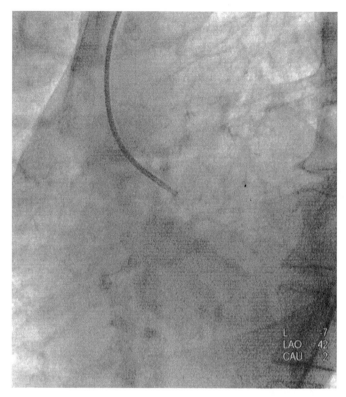

FIGURE 7.10   The multipurpose catheter is shown after clockwise rotation in RAO view.
Note the catheter tip is about 90 degrees from the target of being at the 6-o'clock position.
It must be rotated clockwise from this point.

cause the catheter tip to rise toward the ostium as the catheter is advanced. Occasionally, when the catheter tip hits just above the ostium of the RCA, continued advancement will result in a large, curl-like appearance, and the tip will eventually enter the artery (Figure 7.12). As one advances the catheter, one should be alert to this happening since it can result in successful cannulation of the RCA.

If the RCA is not easily cannulated, its origin most frequently is anteriorly located, though it may be high or even arise anomalously from the left sinus of Valsalva. A RCC shot could be performed to visualize the RCA ostium.

▶ Video 7.7 shows a RCC shot demonstrating the origin of the RCA. High origins may require JR or Amplatz-shaped catheters. As the origin of the RCA becomes more anterior, a JR catheter will not be useful, and the AL or even hockey-stick shape is needed. The

A

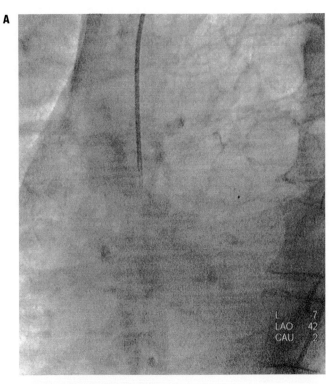

B

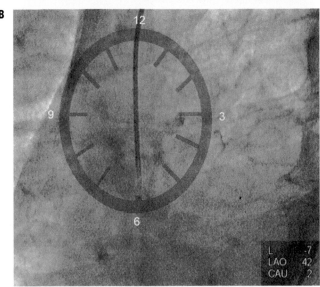

FIGURE 7.11   **Panel A**: The multipurpose catheter is pointing at 6 o'clock in LAO view. It is ready to be advanced in the RCC to assume a flat loop with the tip pointing toward the ostium of the RCA. **Panel B**: A clock superimposed upon the catheter position indicates the 6-o'clock orientation.

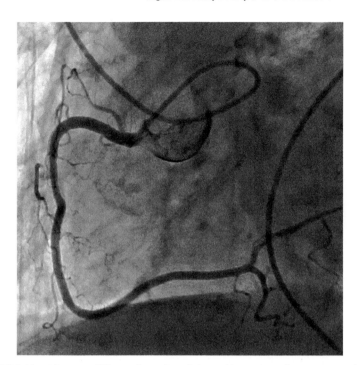

FIGURE 7.12   A large, curl-like configuration of the multipurpose catheter engages the RCA ostium.

first clues to the anomalous origin of the RCA may come when puffs of contrast show an empty sinus with no sign of a RCA. Sometimes, as one rotates the catheter above the aortic valve (the first method of cannulating the RCA), this will result in cannulation of an anomalous circumflex artery. The tip of the JR catheter will sometimes go beyond the ostium of this anomalous vessel and the anomalous circumflex will be entirely missed. Injecting as one pulls the multipurpose catheter back can help in identifying the presence of this anomaly (Figure 7.13).

After LAO, RAO, and perhaps superior views are obtained, the catheter can be withdrawn. It is noteworthy that the superior or frontal-cranial view is very helpful in assessing the distal RCA. It is recommended to observe the multipurpose catheter being removed since withdrawal often results in the catheter going down the artery. One may think that the catheter is out of the artery, yet find that it is even further down the vessel. If there is a lesion in the proximal portion of the RCA, the catheter may move into and disturb the plaque.

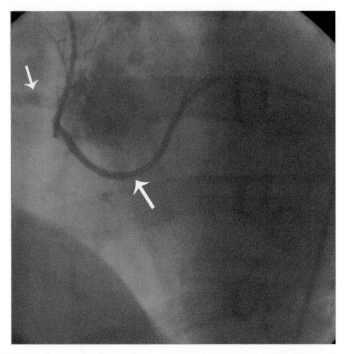

FIGURE 7.13 The multipurpose catheter engages the ostium of an anomalous circumflex artery. The RCA is very close to this position being slightly superior and rotated clockwise from this position. This vessel can be overlooked if the tip of this catheter, or especially a JR catheter, enters the RCA with the tip beyond this ostium.

Left Coronary Artery (LCA) Cannulation

The LCA is cannulated in the RAO view by first rotating the catheter counterclockwise to the NCC (Figure 7.14).

The catheter tip should point posterior as it lies in the NCC. At this point, with the left hand holding the catheter about an inch from the hub of the sheath, the operator should torque the catheter one-half turn clockwise and advance the catheter (Figure 7.15A). As it is advanced, the tip will turn (flip) up anteriorly toward the ostium of the LCA (Figure 7.15B).

▶ Video 7.8 shows engagement of the LCA with the multipurpose catheter in RAO projection, and ▶ Video 7.9 shows the engagement of the LCA with the multipurpose catheter in RAO projection in another patient. This can be done with the left hand alone while the right hand puffs contrast. The catheter must have

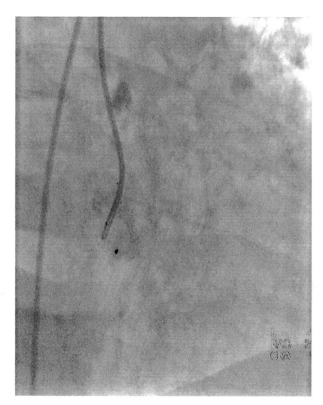

FIGURE 7.14 The multipurpose catheter is rotated counterclockwise into the NCC. It is poised and ready to be advanced with clockwise rotation toward the LCC and the ostium of the LCA.

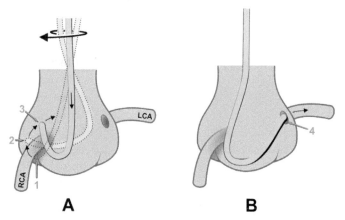

FIGURE 7.15 The following steps are used to cannulate the LCA with a multipurpose catheter. **Panel A**: With the left hand holding the catheter about an inch from the hub of the sheath, the operator torques the catheter one-half turn clockwise and advances the catheter. **Panel B**: As it advances, the tip turns up anteriorly toward the ostium of the LCA.

torque applied such that when advanced in the cusp the torque is transmitted to the tip, resulting in rotation superior and anterior to the region of the LCA. This maneuver can also be done with both hands on the catheter, but generally a single left-hand maneuver is adequate (Figure 7.1A–B). If two hands are required for catheter manipulation, the right hand holds the hub of the catheter with the index finger and thumb and the left hand holds the catheter in a similar fashion. Then the right hand applies about one-half turn of torque to the catheter hub and the left grasps the catheter and advances it in to the NCC. This should result in movement toward the ostium of the LCA (Figure 7.2). When two hands are used and the torque is applied at the hub of the catheter, there are more variables (what happens within the catheter between the hub and the sheath is not a one-to-one action) than are present when the left hand alone does the work. As a result, less success may be achieved in cannulating the LCA when working with two hands.

Often a loop forms and the catheter tip is too far anterior to the LCA ostium (Figure 7.16). In this situation, the catheter is "walked" up posteriorly toward the LCA ostium.

▶ Video 7.10 shows engagement of the LCA with the multipurpose catheter by "walking up the cusp." This is done by applying counterclockwise torsion to the catheter and engaging and disengaging the wall of the LCC. This should result in the catheter tip moving toward the LCA ostium. Too much pushing will result in the catheter tip jumping above the sinotubular ridge such that the process must be started all over again. Based on the catheter tip position, the operator gently advances or retracts the catheter and, if needed, applies minimal clockwise or counterclockwise torque to cannulate the LCA ostium.

Sometimes the LCC can be entered from the right. This is done by placing the catheter in the RCC from the RAO view. With counterclockwise torsion and up-and-down motion, the catheter may jump the commissure into the LCC, at which point it can be "walked up" into the ostium of the LCA (Figure 7.17). Again, as one moves the catheter, care must be taken to avoid advancing the catheter too much in an effort to prevent the catheter from "jumping" above the sinotubular ridge, a position too high in the aorta.

In patients with small aortas, the LCA can sometimes be cannulated by advancing the catheter in the RCC from the RAO view, expecting it to enter the RCA or form a pigtail-like configuration in the aorta (Figure 7.18).

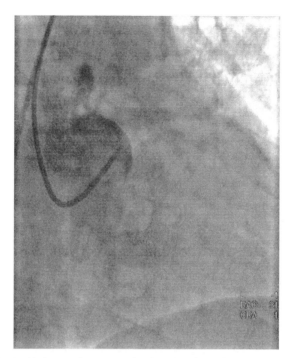

FIGURE 7.16   In this image, the operator is advancing the multipurpose catheter from the NCC to the LCC, but it has landed anterior and below the ostium of the LCA. From this point, the catheter must be "walked up" in a stepwise fashion until it enters the left coronary ostium.

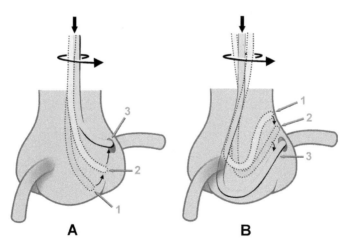

FIGURE 7.17   Steps to cannulate the LCA using a multipurpose catheter. **Panel A**: Applying counterclockwise torsion to the catheter and engaging and disengaging the wall of the LCC results in the catheter tip moving toward the left coronary ostium. **Panel B**: With counterclockwise torsion and up-and-down motion, the catheter jumps the commissure into the left cusp, at which point it can be "walked up" into the ostium of the LCA.

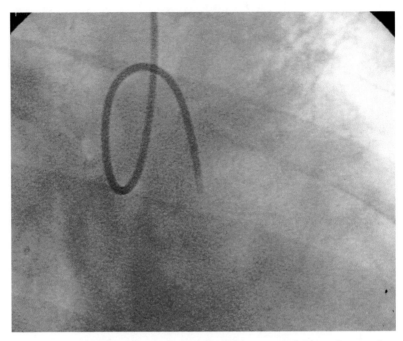

FIGURE 7.18   From this position in the RCC, the multipurpose catheter can be moved to the LCC if rotated counterclockwise, withdrawn slightly, and advanced back down as it uncoils, landing in the LCC.

▶ Video 7.11 shows engagement of the LCA with the multipurpose catheter.

At this point, counterclockwise torsion can be applied and the catheter withdrawn slightly. Subsequently, when a loop forms, it can land in the LCC and be advanced gently in steps up to the ostium of the LCA. On other occasions, when all else fails, the catheter will sometimes land in the LCC when a left ventricle to aorta pullback is done and counterclockwise torsion is applied to the catheter as it is withdrawn.

When a loop is formed in a small aorta and the tip is above the sinotubular ridge, it will usually not drop down into the LCC when withdrawn but almost always falls into the RCC. The best chance of getting the catheter to fall into the LCC is by manipulating the catheter until the tip is pointed directly away from the operator and then gradually withdrawing until it falls down toward the cusp (Figure 7.19). This is the same starting position such that when advanced, the catheter enters the left ventricle. When it drops down, promptly pushing the catheter down can result in upward

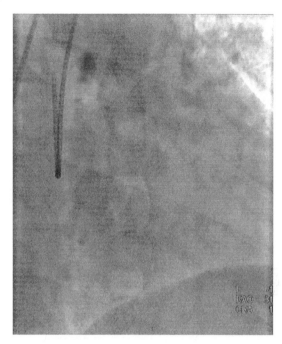

FIGURE 7.19   The image shows the loop of the multipurpose catheter with the tip above the sinotubular ridge. If the aorta is the right size, the catheter can be withdrawn and, as the loop unfolds, it will sometimes fall into the LCC. If clockwise torsion is on the catheter at this point, it will move into the RCC.

motion of the tip toward the ostium of the LCA. This latter move needs to be a rather rapid, downward motion. Although the LCA can frequently be cannulated in patients with small-diameter aortic roots, only a brief period of time should be spent given the ease of using a 3.5-cm curved JL catheter as described in Chapter 6. This is a good general rule concerning the use of the multipurpose catheter. If the artery is not cannulated in a few tries, move on to another catheter. One should not persist for many minutes before something else is tried.

Coronary Bypass Grafts

The multipurpose catheter is a viable option for engaging coronary bypass grafts. The left coronary bypass grafts should be approached from the RAO view (although some prefer the LAO).

▶ Video 7.12 shows engagement of a left coronary bypass graft with the multipurpose catheter in the RAO projection.

▶ Video 7.13 shows engagement of another coronary bypass graft with the multipurpose catheter. The small "o-ring" markers placed by cardiothoracic surgeons on the proximal aortic anastomosis suture line are very helpful in locating the grafts at the time of catheterization.

The lowest left coronary graft on the ascending aorta is the LAD (if the IMA was not used) or diagonal graft followed superiorly by vein grafts that go to ramus or anterior marginals, mid marginals, and then posterior marginals in ascending positions in that order on the aorta. Some surgeons place larger, wire-like rings around the ostium of the saphenous vein origins, making these targets very easy. Less obvious markers are small clips placed adjacent to the origin of the grafts. Some seem not to have any markers (Figure 7.20A–E).

When radial artery or free internal mammary grafts (detached from their subclavian artery origin) are used, their proximal

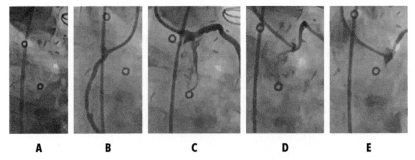

A	**B**	**C**	**D**	**E**

FIGURE 7.20   **Panel A:** The RAO view of the aorta showing two markers for the coronary bypass grafts. The lower marker indicates the position of the right coronary bypass graft on the right side of the aorta. On the opposite side of the aorta (about 130 degrees over toward the left side of the aorta) and in a higher position, the other marker indicates the highest of the left coronary bypass grafts. **Panel B:** The multipurpose catheter has been rotated counterclockwise until it has engaged the right coronary bypass graft. **Panel C:** The highest of the saphenous vein grafts (on the opposite side of the aorta from the right coronary bypass graft) is engaged by clockwise rotation of the multipurpose catheter. This bypass graft usually goes to a posterior marginal branch of the left circumflex artery. **Panel D:** The catheter has been removed from the upper graft by counterclockwise rotation, pushed down, and then rotated clockwise to the position of the next saphenous vein graft, which is typically the mid obtuse marginal vessel graft. **Panel E:** The catheter is rotated counterclockwise out of the mid obtuse marginal graft, pushed down, and then clocked around into the lower saphenous vein graft, which is usually the diagonal vessel graft. This completes the right coronary bypass graft on the right side of the aorta and the three left coronary bypass grafts on the opposite side of the aorta.

anastomosis to the aortic wall, side of a vein graft, or trunk of an in-situ LIMA may not be obvious from markers. It is important to have this information if possible before starting the procedure. It will avoid a lot of searching around, reduce radiation, and save a lot of contrast. This is particularly important if the patient has renal insufficiency.

Although the above-described locations of grafts on the aorta are the norm, sometimes there are variations. The site of vein graft anastomoses may vary by surgeon's preference or, more importantly, to avoid atherosclerotic disease and calcification in the proximal ascending aorta. At the time of catheterization before the surgical procedure, it is good to note the presence of calcium in the ascending aorta and point this out to the surgeon. Sometimes the calcification is so severe (i.e., "eggshell aortas") that the procedure cannot be safely done. Cross clamping of the aorta or punching the holes for the proximal anastomosis can result in aortic dissection. Once these positions have been identified, the multipurpose catheter can be rotated clockwise while watching for the catheter tip to engage usually the lowest graft first or whatever is found. Puffs of contrast help in locating these origins.

When rotating the catheter clockwise, slightly moving the catheter up and down will transfer the torque to the tip, allowing it to move in small increments. Once a graft origin is engaged and a puff of contrast indicates such, slight forward pressure is applied to stabilize the catheter. Sometimes the clockwise torsion needs to be removed by slightly rotating counterclockwise such that the catheter is neutral from the torque standpoint. This will stabilize the catheter such that when injected, the catheter will not move out of position.

Once the catheter is stable, injection of the saphenous vein graft (SVG) can be done. Sometimes when only a "stump" of a SVG remains, a "drive-by" shot can be done just to document the occlusion. After the first SVG is engaged, the catheter can be moved superiorly by rotating counterclockwise, pulling up, and then rotating clockwise back to the SVG above. This procedure can be repeated until all of the left SVGs are engaged and injected. It is important to know the exact number of grafts for which one is searching and whether branching vein grafts ("Y grafts") or multi-anastomotic, sequential vein grafts ("snake grafts") are present. When the native circulation is examined, one should look for competitive flow indicating the presence of a bypass graft. Also, occluded grafts often leave their mark on the grafted vessel as areas of "tenting" or small segments of SVGs that remain like a small diverticulum on the vessel. In patients with prior bypass surgery, it is important to make absolutely sure that each myocardial segment is supplied by a native coronary or grafted vessel. "Gaps" in coverage suggest that a bypass graft or native vessel has not been injected.

The saphenous vein bypass grafts on the right side of the aorta are best engaged by applying counterclockwise torque to the catheter from the NCC. The RAO view is usually preferred.

▶ Video 7.14 shows engagement of a right coronary bypass graft with the multipurpose catheter in the RAO projection. The take-off of the SVG to the RCA may be quite posteriorly located.

Slight up-and-down motion of the catheter tip as one applies counterclockwise torque with the left hand at the sheath hub will usually result in engagement of the ostium of the SVG to the RCA.

▶ Video 7.15 shows engagement of an occluded right coronary bypass graft with the multipurpose catheter in LAO projection.

As one first starts using the multipurpose catheter, the left hand should be holding the catheter close to the hub of the sheath and the right hand at the hub of the catheter. The left hand should be the primary operating hand, with torque placed on the catheter between the thumb and index fingers and the right hand at the hub helping the left hand with rotation of the catheter.

Occasionally, as one approaches the subclavian artery to inject the IMA, the angle of the IMA catheter is too acute to turn up into the ostium of the subclavian artery. The multipurpose catheter can be used to engage the subclavian and to introduce the wire into the artery. A flush injection can be made to identify the IMA and sometimes get enough information to establish patency. If not, an exchange wire can be used to place the IMA catheter up into the subclavian and engage the IMA to make direct injections. Renal arteries can also be partially engaged and located using the multipurpose catheter and injected in a "drive-by" fashion.

The multipurpose catheter can also be used to cross the aortic valve. The catheter is used in conjunction with a straight wire without a movable tip. The usual up-and-down motion of the wire along with rotation of the catheter tip is often successful in getting the wire to cross the valve. Although the LAO view is most helpful, the RAO view can also be used.

Challenging Conditions

A number of challenging conditions require special techniques. These include:

- Small aortic root
- Tortuous iliac arteries, as seen in the elderly
- Large aortic root
- Tortuous and large descending aorta
- Diseased iliac vessels that bind the catheter
- Short stature
- Individuals with long trunks (may require 125-cm multipurpose catheter)
- Anomalous origin of each coronary artery

Each of the above-listed challenges has specific solutions. The small aortic root requires a Judkins technique in general. Tortuous iliac arteries can be overcome by using a long Arrow sheath to straighten out to some degree the curves in the artery, as described in Chapter 5. One must watch for catheter kinking, especially when the catheter is vigorously rotated. When this occurs, the pressure damps and the groin must be visualized. The catheter should be rotated in the opposite direction until the kinking is no longer present. Large aortic roots are very difficult, and the multipurpose catheter should be manipulated gently to limit the risk of perforating or dissecting the aorta. The tortuous large descending aorta is difficult with a multipurpose catheter, and bailing out to the Judkins technique should be done early. Very tortuous iliac vessels and the binding that they have on the catheter can be lessened with a long Arrow sheath. If binding of the catheter persists, use of a sheath one French size larger than the catheter can sometimes be helpful. Smaller individuals are difficult and often require a JL 3.5-cm curve to get to the LCA. Taller individuals with long trunks may require a longer catheter when the hub of the catheter is up to the sheath. Anomalous coronaries require a careful look to ensure a vessel supplies all segments of the left ventricle. If the multipurpose catheter does not do the job, catheters like the Amplatz are useful.

As skills develop with the multipurpose catheter, more and more patients can be done entirely by this single-catheter technique. If, however, the coronary artery is not successfully cannulated with the multipurpose catheter in a few tries, move on to another catheter. The use of the multipurpose catheter is a constant learning process.

References

1. Schoonmaker FW, King SB. Coronary arteriography by the single catheter percutaneous femoral technique. Experience in 6800 cases. *Circulation.* 1974;50:735-740.

2. King SB, Douglas JS. *Coronary arteriography and angioplasty.* New York: McGraw-Hill; 1984.

3. Clements SD, Gatlin S. Outpatient cardiac catheterization: a report of 3,000 cases. *Clin Cardiol.* 1991;14(6):477-480.

Video Legends

Video 7.1 Left ventriculography with the MP catheter; RAO projection

Video 7.2 Left ventriculography with the MP catheter; LAO projection

Video 7.3 Incorrect position of the MP catheter for left ventriculography

Video 7.4 Engaging the RCA with the MP catheter; RAO projection

Video 7.5 Engaging the RCA with the MP catheter; RAO projection

Video 7.6 Using the MP catheter to cannulate the RCA; LAO projection

Video 7.7 RCC shot showing the RCA

Video 7.8 Engaging the LCA with the MP catheter; RAO projection

Video 7.9 Engaging the LCA with the MP catheter; RAO projection

Video 7.10 Engaging the LCA with the MP catheter; "walking up the cusp"

Video 7.11 Engaging the LCA with the MP catheter

Video 7.12 Engaging a left coronary bypass graft with the MP catheter; RAO projection

Video 7.13 Engaging a coronary bypass graft with the MP catheter

Video 7.14 Engaging a right coronary bypass graft with the MP catheter; RAO projection

Video 7.15 Engaging an occluded right coronary bypass graft with the MP catheter; LAO projection

CHAPTER 8

Angiography of Coronary Bypass Grafts

"Never assume something which you have not seen proof of."

—Anonymous

Venous and Free Arterial Grafts

Before proceeding with cardiac catheterization, it is important to review the previous catheterization images and reports if available. Surgical reports and catheterization images will help the operator to choose the right strategy and reduce the length and the risk of the procedure. Most cardiothoracic surgeons leave a specific marker close to the site of the venous graft anastomosis on the aorta to mark the origin of the graft, as described in Chapter 7. The position of surgical clips might also simplify the search for the origin of the vein graft. Another tip comes from angiography of the native coronaries: the absence of collateral or native coronary flow to a segment of myocardium that still contracts suggests the presence of patent graft blood supply. Occasionally, retrograde filling of the graft may point to the site of graft origin.

Surgical placement of vein grafts follows certain rules: the proximal anastomosis of the left coronary vein grafts are placed very close together vertically or horizontally on the left anterior surface of the ascending aorta (right silhouetted border of the aorta on the imaging screen in the RAO and LAO projections), and on the right anterior surface (left silhouetted border of the aorta on the imaging screen in the RAO and LAO projections) for right coronary grafts (Figure 8.1). The obtuse marginal grafts may be attached to the

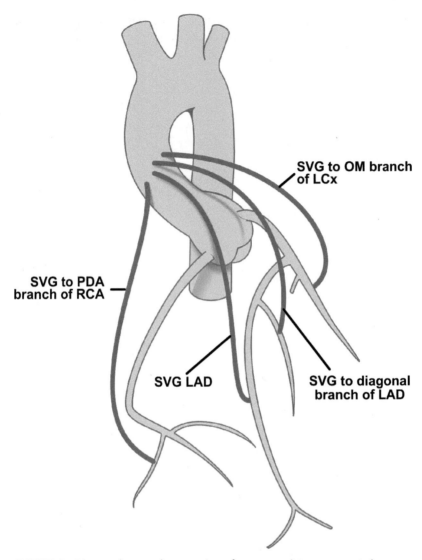

SVG to OM branch of LCx

SVG to PDA branch of RCA

SVG LAD

SVG to diagonal branch of LAD

FIGURE 8.1   Diagram shows saphenous vein grafts to appropriate coronary arteries.

posterior surface of the aorta, and may require an AL catheter for easy cannulation of their ostia. In general, vein grafts to the RCA are located most inferiorly followed by grafts to the LAD, diagonals and obtuse marginal branches of the LCX.

In each individual case, the choice of the first catheter can vary; a JR coronary catheter may be used initially to catheterize all saphenous vein grafts. The bypass grafts can be cannulated after native coronary vessel catheterization is completed. Angiography of the native coronary arteries can provide important information about the bypass grafts. For example, the presence of extensive collateral blood flow from the other arteries to the artery subserved by the graft suggests the presence of hemodynamically significant stenosis or occlusion in the graft; retrograde filling of the entire graft or presence of competitive distal blood flow indicates an open graft, and on the contrary, normal distal flow in the bypassed native vessel without graft filling and without competitive flow may suggest that the graft is closed.

Attempts to cannulate saphenous vein grafts[1] start after the operator finishes obtaining the angiographic images of the native coronary arteries. Then under fluoroscopic guidance in 45-degree LAO view, the tip of the JR catheter is gently moved back from the ostium of the RCA without rotation. The catheter tip first hangs onto the ostium of the RCA, extends, and then after leaving the coronary ostium and returning to its natural curve, may cannulate the origin of one of the vein grafts. If this maneuver is unsuccessful, the process of graft-seeking continues by gently moving the catheter up and down in the ascending aorta with slight clockwise or counterclockwise rotation.

Certain rules apply to this process:

1. Most vein grafts will be located in the projection between the second and forth sternal sutures.
2. Ostia of the grafts usually will be close to the surgical clips or specific surgical markers.
3. Grafts to the RCA are best engaged in LAO 45-degree projection, while grafts to the LCA are best cannulated in RAO 30-degree projection.
4. The tip of the catheter, when coaxially cannulating the ostium of the right venous graft in 45-degree LAO view, is oriented to the patient's right; when coaxially cannulating the ostium of the left venous graft in 30-degree RAO view, the tip of the catheter is also oriented to the patient's right. On the other hand, when the tip of the catheter is coaxially cannulating the ostium of the right vein graft in 30-degree RAO view, it is oriented to the patient's left, and when the tip of the catheter is coaxially cannulating the ostium of the left vein graft in 45-degree LAO view, it is also oriented to the patient's left.
5. If the catheter tip is not moving freely, causing the body of the catheter to buckle with gentle advancement, the operator should stop maneuvering the catheter, observe the pressure curve, and if fine, proceed with a small test injection of contrast.

6. It is recommended to rotate clockwise and slightly advance the catheter body when its tip is positioned slightly above the anticipated location of the graft ostium, since clockwise rotation moves the tip caudally, and slight forward movement fixes the tip in the ostium of the vein graft.
7. The tip of the catheter should be placed coaxially in the ostium of the graft to avoid deep engagement with damping of the pressure waveform.
8. If the ostium of the left bypass graft is not found with the JR, or when the JR catheter does not reach the anterior wall of the aorta where the left coronary bypass grafts' origins are located, or the tip of the catheter cannot be adequately aligned with the ostium of the superiorly oriented vein graft, other catheters should be tried (Table 8.1).

    If the operator is not successful in cannulating the bypass graft, biplane ascending aortography in LAO and RAO projections should be performed before concluding that the bypass grafts are occluded. Even the absence of graft opacification on biplane aortography is not 100% specific for occluded grafts.
9. Once the graft is safely cannulated, LAO and RAO angiographic views are obtained. Additional projections can be obtained if an operator wants to specifically look at the distal anastomosis; for grafts to obtuse marginal branches of the left circumflex artery: 30-degree RAO caudal 30-degree, or AP caudal 45-degree; for left anterior descending: 30-degree RAO 30-degree cranial, or AP 45-degree cranial, or 45-degree LAO 30-degree cranial, or left lateral; for diagonal branches of the LAD: AP 45-degree

TABLE 8.1   Catheters used in coronary bypass graft cannulation.

Right Coronary Bypass Grafts:
- Multipurpose catheter
- Right coronary bypass catheter
- Modified Amplatz right catheter
- 3-DRCA
- Amplatz left catheter

Left Coronary Bypass Grafts:
- Left coronary bypass catheter
- Multipurpose catheter
- Amplatz left catheter (especially in superiorly oriented saphenous vein grafts and grafts placed high in the ascending aorta)
- Modified Amplatz right catheter
- Internal mammary catheter

cranial, or 45-degree LAO 30-degree cranial; and for posterior descending and posterolateral branches of the RCA: 30-degree RAO 30-degree cranial, or AP 45-degree cranial, or 45-degree LAO 30-degree cranial.

10. The operator should avoid performing angiography with the tip of the catheter sitting deep in the graft since ostial stenosis could be missed. If the tip of the diagnostic catheter is not coaxially aligned with the bypass graft, the graft may be called stenotic since the ostium can be directed inferiorly or superiorly and not opacify with injection.

With the left brachial or radial approaches, the operator uses the long exchange J-tip guidewire to exchange the JR to any other catheter needed to successfully cannulate the graft. Subsequent steps are identical to the ones described above and in the previous chapters. Bypass graft vessel perforation is extremely rare with diagnostic catheterization and mostly is seen in interventional practice. Management depends on the severity of bleeding and the use of antiplatelet and anticoagulant agents, periprocedurally. Perfusion balloons, covered stents and emergent surgery are potential treatment options

Pediculed Arterial Grafts

When performing angiography of brachiocephalic and subclavian arteries,[1] it is recommended to use nonionic contrast in order to decrease the risk of neurotoxicity and arm discomfort caused by ionic high-osmolar contrast dye. The JR coronary catheter or IMA catheter can be used to successfully cannulate both right and left IMAs (Figure 8.2). To engage the brachiocephalic trunk the JR catheter is placed in the distal segment of the ascending aorta in a 45-degree LAO or PA projection. Under fluoroscopic guidance, the operator slowly torques the catheter counterclockwise as a unit. This is accomplished by slow, step-by-step (half-turn), counterclockwise rotations. After each turn, a small amount of time is allowed for transmission of the torque applied at the base of the catheter to its tip, just enough to point the catheter tip towards the patient's head. To facilitate the transmission of torque to the tip of the catheter, sometimes minimal in-and-out movement of the catheter is performed. The step-wise rotation allows the operator

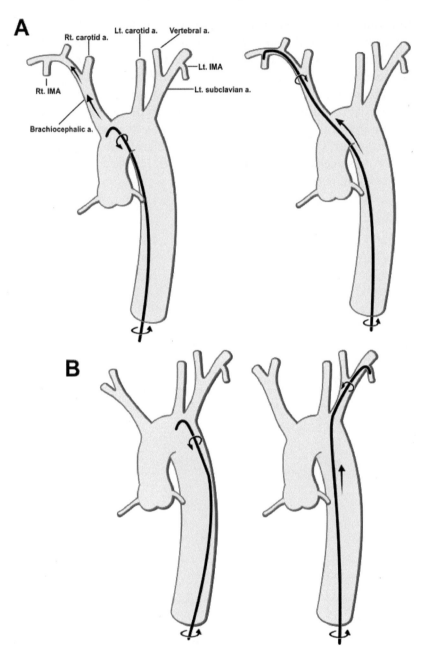

FIGURE 8.2 Drawings showing selective cannulation of the RIMA (**Panel A**) and LIMA (**Panel B**) (see text for details).

to avoid over-torqueing the catheter tip and flipping it around in the aortic arch. As soon as the tip is appropriately positioned, the catheter is slowly pulled back until its tip "dives" into the brachiocephalic artery. This can be easily noticed by observing the sudden movement of the tip up into the aortic arch, as if the tip of the catheter prolapses into a hole. When this occurs and the right internal mammary artery (RIMA) is the target of investigation, a test injection of about 5–6 mL of contrast material in PA projection is performed in order to rule out brachiocephalic and/or right subclavian stenosis and severe tortuosity. This test injection will also orient the operator to the position of the tip of the catheter and the neighboring arteries, since in some cases the tip of the catheter ends up deep in the right subclavian artery in close proximity to the RIMA, or the RIMA may arise from the brachiocephalic artery itself before the ostium of the right subclavian artery. If the tip of the catheter accidentally ends up just beyond the origin of the RIMA, the operator slowly torques the catheter clockwise, bringing the tip anterior, since IMAs arise anteroinferiorly. If over-torqueing occurs, a gentle reverse turn usually takes care of the problem.

Several test injections under fluoroscopy for better orientation may precede the cannulation of the artery. As soon as the tip is appropriately positioned, the catheter is slowly pulled back until the tip of the catheter "snags" the ostium of the RIMA. When this occurs, the operator applies a half-turn of counterclockwise torque to eliminate the tension of the earlier applied clockwise torque and checks the pressure tracing; if normal, the operator performs a test injection of contrast to assure the coaxial position of its tip in the ostium of the IMA in order to avoid arterial dissection, to which IMAs are predisposed. Emergent stent placement is the way to manage this complication if discovered in a timely manner. Occasionally, the patient may be asked to turn his/her head to the left or to the right and breathe in or out to facilitate engagement of the RIMA ostium. Once this is done, the operator initiates angiography in LAO and RAO cranial views, comes off pressure, and injects 6–8 mL of the contrast dye into the artery under an initially slow rise, but subsequently steady and with constant pressure to opacify the vessel lumen and to avoid streaming of contrast material.

In general with RIMA catheterization, the tip of the catheter initially ends up in the origin of the brachiocephalic artery proximal to the ostium of the RIMA, requiring the use of a long exchange J-tip guidewire. A guidewire is advanced through the catheter to the brachiocephalic artery, using a small turn of the catheter tip to avoid the right common carotid artery, and placed deep into the right subclavian artery. This is followed by exchange of the JR to an IMA catheter over the wire and advancement of the IMA catheter over the guidewire under fluoroscopic guidance into the right subclavian artery. When the catheter is placed in the distal segment of the right subclavian artery, the guidewire is removed. The process for cannulating the RIMA is identical to the one described with the JR catheter. After angiography is completed, a counterclockwise rotation of the catheter disengages its tip from the RIMA ostium and the operator moves the catheter back into the aortic arch.

To engage the left subclavian artery, the JR or IMA catheter is placed in the distal segment of the ascending aorta in 45-degree LAO or PA projection as described above. As soon as the tip is appropriately positioned the catheter is slowly pulled back. First, the tip of the catheter gets into the brachiocephalic artery as described above. Once this occurs, withdrawal of the catheter continues. The catheter returns to the aorta, and upon further withdrawal, gets into the left common carotid artery. Gentle pull-back continues until the catheter again returns to the aorta and subsequently gets into the left subclavian artery. When this occurs, test injections in PA or LAO position similar to the one described above for the brachiocephalic artery are performed to orient the operator to the placement of the catheter tip and to the tortuosity of the proximal left subclavian artery, to exclude subclavian stenosis, and to potentially visualize the origin of the LIMA. In case of significant tortuosity of the proximal left subclavian artery, angiography should be performed in RAO 30-degree projection (LAO 30-degree for RIMA), to better assess the tortuosity of the vessel. After angiographic images of the proximal left subclavian artery are obtained, the operator returns the camera to the PA position, the hub of the catheter gets disconnected from the manifold, a 5- to 10-mL syringe is attached, and 1–2 mL of blood is aspirated. A long exchange J-tip guidewire is carefully advanced through the catheter into the distal left subclavian artery followed by the JR exchange to IMA catheter over the guidewire. After the guidewire is withdrawn, the catheter will be attached to the manifold and pressure checked; the operator slowly torques the catheter counterclockwise under fluoroscopy, bringing the tip anteriorly. As soon as the tip is appropriately positioned, the catheter is slowly pulled back until the tip of the catheter "snags" the ostium of the LIMA. For better orientation, several test injections under fluoroscopy may precede the cannulation of the ostium of the artery. When this occurs, the operator checks the pressure tracings and, if normal, performs a test injection of contrast dye to assure a coaxial position of its tip in the ostium of the LIMA. Only after these precautions is angiography performed in PA and left lateral projections. If the left lateral projection cannot be done, a straight 30-degree RAO view or 30-degree RAO with 20-degree caudal angulation view can be used to visualize the distal anastomosis.

After completion of angiography, the catheter tip is gently removed from the ostium of the LIMA under fluoroscopic guidance by slow, step-by-step (half-turn), clockwise rotation of the catheter. The operator moves the catheter back into the descending aorta only after making sure that the catheter tip has disengaged from the LIMA ostium. If the LIMA originates from the vertical portion of the subclavian artery, diagnostic catheters such as JR or Bernstein (AngioDynamics, Inc., Latham, NY) are more successful in cannulating the vessel.

An alternative approach for left subclavian cannulation is a proximal approach to it from the descending segment of the aortic arch. With this method, the IMA catheter is placed over the J-tip, 0.035-inch guidewire; the wire tip is moved back to hide about one-quarter of an inch from the tip of the catheter in order to allow greater flexibility of the tip as it approaches the left subclavian artery, where a gentle counterclockwise rotation with slight advancement allows the catheter tip to enter the ostium of the artery. Subsequent steps are identical to the ones described above.

When a brachial or radial approach is taken to cannulate the RIMA or LIMA, the operator uses the appropriate side for access, since RIMA usually is not approached and cannulated from the left arm, and vice versa. On the other hand, when approached through the appropriate arm, cannulation of the arterial grafts usually is easy. The J-tip, 0.035-inch guidewire is introduced through the arterial sheath, and the tip positioned in the proximal segment of the left or right subclavian artery. This is followed by placement of the IMA catheter over the wire and subsequent wire removal. The catheter is flushed with normal saline and the subclavian pressure is monitored, followed by a test injection under fluoroscopic guidance in order to orient the operator to the position of the tip of the catheter and neighboring arteries. Subsequently, the operator retrieves the catheter slowly and applies a slow, step-by-step (half-turn) rotation, using clockwise torque for the LIMA and counterclockwise for the RIMA. As soon as the tip is appropriately positioned, the catheter is slowly pulled back until the tip of the catheter "snags" the ostium of the IMA. The rest of the steps have been described above.

In rare clinical scenarios the angiographer faces the need to cannulate the LIMA from the right-arm access.[2] In order to accomplish this task, the left subclavian artery should be cannulated first. To do this, the Simmons sidewinder catheter (AngioDynamics, Inc.) should be used, but if not available, a left or right coronary bypass catheter can be substituted. After the subclavian artery is cannulated, the Simmons catheter is exchanged over the exchange long J-tip, 0.035-inch guidewire to an IMA catheter for selective cannulation of the LIMA ostium.

In cases when the RIMA and LIMA cannot be selectively engaged, the catheter should be placed in close vicinity to the appropriate artery, and a blood pressure cuff inflated on the corresponding arm above systolic blood pressure (to direct contrast preferentially to the proximal branches of the subclavian artery) for nonselective angiography.[3] Nonselective subclavian artery angiography is also performed in patients with symptoms of subclavian steal syndrome.

Other arterial grafts usually used by cardiothoracic surgeons are free RIMA and LIMA, radial and right gastroepiploic arteries. The approach to free RIMA, LIMA, and radial arteries is analogous to the standard approach to SVGs described earlier. These grafts are smaller in diameter compared to vein grafts. The important point to remember when interrogating the free radial artery graft is its tendency towards spasm, so it is advised to inject 100 mcg of nitroglycerin selectively into the graft prior to graft angiography. The right gastroepiploic arterial graft is usually attached to the right or left PDA. This artery is a branch of the hepatic artery, which originates from the celiac trunk. To cannulate the hepatic artery, the operator usually uses a 4-Fr Cobra catheter and cannulates the celiac trunk first utilizing the left lateral view. The benefit of using this view is better visualization of the ostium of the celiac trunk. The long exchange hydrophilic wire is run carefully through the 4-Fr Cobra catheter and is navigated through the celiac trunk and hepatic artery into the right gastroepiploic artery, where it gets fixed. To help with maneuvering the slippery guidewire, a stopcock is placed on the tail of the wire and locked. This stopcock can be used as a steering wheel and assists the operator in performing rotational movements of the guidewire when interrogating the branching artery. When the guidewire is finally positioned into the right gastroepiploic artery the 4-Fr Cobra catheter is exchanged for a Bernstein catheter, and the guidewire is removed. After successful cannulation of the right gastroepiploic artery, the operator initiates angiography in LAO and RAO cranial views. When all appropriate angiographic images are obtained, the proximal end of the catheter gets disconnected from the manifold, and the operator advances the J-tip guidewire through the catheter into the right gastroepiploic artery under fluoroscopic guidance until the tip of the wire protrudes beyond the tip of the catheter. This is followed by simultaneous catheter and wire removal from the body through the arterial sheath.

References

1. Casserly IP, Messenger JC. Technique and catheters. *Cardiol Clin.* 2009;27:417-432.
2. Cha KS, Kim MH. Feasibility and safety of concomitant left internal mammary arteriography at the setting of the right transradial coronary angiography. *Cathet Cardiovasc Intervent.* 2002;56:188-195.
3. Bhatt SN, Jorgensen MB, Aharonian VJ, Mahrer PR. Nonselective angiography of the internal mammary artery: a fast, reliable, and safe technique. *Cathet Cardiovasc Diagn.* 1995;36:194-198.

CHAPTER 9

Left and Right Ventriculography, Aortography, and Pulmonary Angiography

"It's not what you look at that matters, it's what you see."

—Henry David Thoreau

Radiologic Anatomy of the Heart and Left Ventriculography

The angiographer performing left and right cardiac catheterization should be familiar not only with the cardiac structures in general, but primarily the projections of those cardiac structures in different angiographic views.[1,2] Left heart structures are outlined in different projections in Figures 9.1 and 9.2.

Measuring left ventricular (LV) pressure with or without accompanied ventriculography is a routine part of any left heart catheterization procedure.

The general indications for LV catheterization are:

1. Measuring LV end diastolic pressure
2. Establishing presence of and measuring aortic valve, LV outflow, or intracavitary gradients

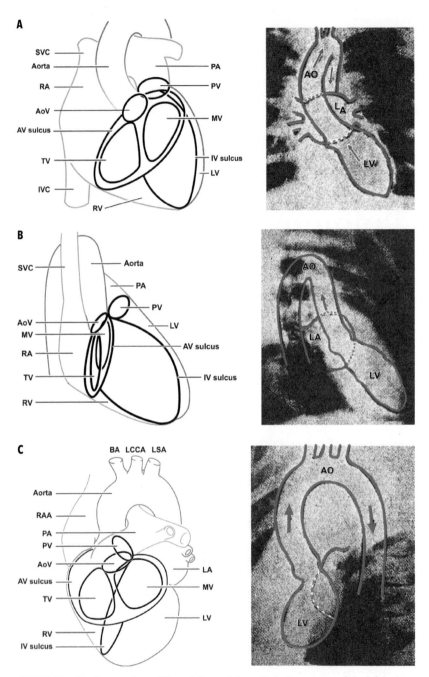

FIGURE 9.1 The images show different views of the radiologic anatomy of the left heart and aorta with corresponding diagram. **Panel A**: PA view; **Panel B**: RAO view; **Panel C**: LAO view; **Panel D**: LL view.

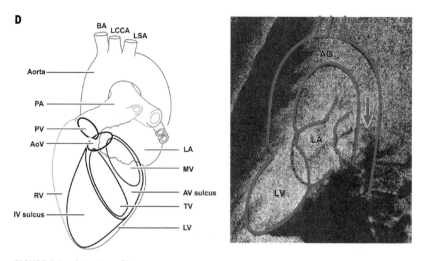

FIGURE 9.1 (*Continued*)

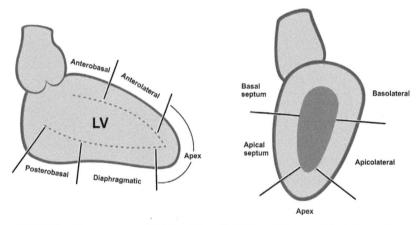

FIGURE 9.2 Diagrams show RAO (**Panel A**) and LAO (**Panel B**) views of the left ventricle.

3. Assessing LV systolic function, presence of segmental wall motion abnormalities and myocardial viability (noted by postextrasystolic contractile augmentation)
4. Assessing severity of mitral regurgitation
5. Establishing presence and severity of ventricular septal defects

If LV end-diastolic pressure exceeds 25 mmHg, it is generally recommended not to perform left ventriculography unless the pressure is reduced by intravenous diuretics or sublingual nitroglycerin.

Certain restrictions and contraindications to the procedure are listed in Table 9.1.

TABLE 9.1   Contraindications to left ventriculography.

- Mechanical aortic valve prosthesis
- Active aortic valve and/or mitral valve endocarditis
- LV mobile mass
- LV fresh thrombus
- LV old apical thrombus*
- Decompensated heart failure**
- Severe aortic stenosis**
- Severe left main coronary stenosis**

* relative contraindication for ventriculography and pressure measurement
** absolute contraindication for ventriculography, no contraindication for pressure measurement

Entering the Left Ventricle

When planning to cross a severely stenotic aortic valve and antic-ipating difficulty, it is advised to give intravenous heparin bolus and keep the ACT above 200 seconds during the procedure. The guidewire should be removed and cleaned every 2 minutes and the catheters aspirated and flushed before every attempt to thread the guidewire.

THE ANGLED PIGTAIL CATHETER

The angled pigtail catheter (depicted in Chapter 3, Figure 3.8) is specifically designed to enter the LV and to prevent the tip of the catheter from aggressively contacting the endocardial surface. The distal tip of this catheter has 6 side holes to allow the rapid filling of the ventricular cavity with contrast and to avoid an excessive motion of the catheter in the LV during the injection phase. The operator advances the catheter over the 0.035-inch, J-tip guidewire through the arterial sheath to the aorta under fluoroscopic guid-ance, keeping the tip of the wire protruding beyond the tip of the catheter. Once the tip of the guidewire advances around the aortic arch, it gets fixed above the sinotubular junction. The catheter slides over the wire, and the wire is withdrawn. In 30-degree RAO projec-tion, the catheter is rotated in the ascending aorta until the "pigtail" tip looks like the number "6" and oriented towards the left cusp. When this is achieved, the operator slowly advances the catheter towards the aortic valve. Occasionally, the catheter tip easily pro-lapses into the ventricular cavity, but frequently it gets caught by the aortic valve cusps. In such cases, a gentle push of the catheter will cause buckling of its distal end. Slow withdrawal with a slight clockwise rotation of the catheter straightens the distal segment, and the patient is asked to take a deep breath. With this maneuver, the catheter tip usually prolapses into the LV cavity, where it gets stabilized in the mid-ventricular position coaxial with the longitudinal axis of the LV. The LV systolic and end-diastolic pressures are measured and recorded on 200-mm and 50-mm scales on end-expiration. Once this is done, the operator fills the syringe with contrast and proceeds with a test injection into the LV cavity under fluoroscopic guidance in order to optimize catheter position and ensure that it is not lying against the LV wall or entrapped in the mitral valve apparatus, as described in Chapter 7.

If an atypical anatomic configuration, sclero-calcific changes of the aortic valve, or the use of small, 4-Fr or 5-Fr diameter catheters impedes the process of crossing the valve with the above-described method, one of the following techniques using guidewire support can be applied. First, the catheter slides over the 0.035-inch, J-tip guidewire until the tip of the wire gets covered by the tip of the catheter and the guidewire stays inside the catheter. The rest of the technique is identical to the one described earlier. Second, initial steps are the same as in the previous approach until the "pigtail" tip looks like the number "6." At this point, the guidewire is advanced forward against the valve. Sometimes the guidewire slips straight across the valve, but if not, the operator gently pushes it forward until 3–4 cm of the distal end is buckled and curled back in the aortic sinus just as described above. Then the catheter is withdrawn slightly, followed by gentle withdrawal of the wire. When the curve of the guidewire straightens, it usually prolapses through the valve. If the tip of the catheter is placed too deep into the LV and/or twists with each beat, then it may be entangled in the subvalvular apparatus and requires repositioning.

While monitoring the LV pressure and ECG, the injector syringe is disconnected from the manifold, which then is connected to a power injector. To perform this maneuver safely, the technician manually runs contrast media through the tubing system connected to the injector until contrast is ejected from the distal tip of the tubing. At the same time, the operator allows the contrast from the bottle to run down through the manifold by opening the proximal port of the manifold. Then the operator hooks the distal end of the tubing from the injector to the manifold by using the fluid-to-fluid method. If some air has managed to remain in the tubing, gently tapping on the tubing with simultaneous aspiration of the air bubbles into the injector takes care of it. About 8–10 mL of blood from the LV is aspirated back into the automatic contrast injector, while the operator taps gently on the tubing and manifold in order to remove all bubbles before moving the contrast forward into the ventricle for test injection under fluoroscopy guidance. The injector filled with the contrast is positioned at 80 to 90 degrees so all the potentially present air bubbles in the closed system collect on the top surface of the dye, preventing their migration into the ventricle during the injection. After this step is completed and another check for the absence of air from the system is performed, the operator sets the final parameters for injection.

Once the catheter is sitting properly in the mid ventricle, the physician will inform the patient that he/she may feel a hot flush all over the body and the sensation of passing urine. Then the patient is asked to hold a breath while the operator takes the image and fixes the catheter at the hub of the sheath to prevent backward recoil, and orders contrast injection. Imaging in 60-degree LAO and 30-degree RAO projections is initiated and ventriculography is performed. Ventriculography should continue until the ventricle is clear of contrast.

The usual settings of the power injector for left ventriculography are 30–50 mL of contrast dye volume at an injection rate of 12–15 mL/second and gradual flow rate rise over 0.5–1.0 second when a 6-Fr pigtail catheter is used. The frame rate is set at 15 frames/second unless the patient is tachycardic. In such cases, the frame rate is set at 30 frames/second. These parameters and radiologic views vary based on individual patient characteristics and the purpose of the study. Large volume (50 mL) and high rates (15–20 mL/sec) of injection are needed with a dilated ventricle, in a patient with high cardiac output, or when assessing severity of mitral regurgitation (Table 9.2). In general, views for evaluation of severity of mitral regurgitation in biplane ventriculography are RAO 45-degree and LAO 60-degree with 25-degree cranial angulation, since these projections place the left atrium away from the spine, the left ventricle,

TABLE 9.2 Angiographic classification of mitral regurgitation severity.

1. Mild (1+) - Minimal and incomplete opacification of the left atrium, which clears with each cardiac cycle
2. Moderate (2+) - Complete but faint opacification of the left atrium after several cardiac cycles
3. Moderate to Severe (3+) - Complete opacification of the left atrium after more than one cardiac cycle, with the same intensity as left ventricle
4. Severe (4+) - Complete and very intense opacification of the left atrium within one cardiac cycle, with opacification of pulmonary veins

and the descending aorta. The patient's heart rate should be well controlled, since severity of mitral regurgitation cannot be adequately evaluated in patients with tachycardia, frequent premature contractions, or uncontrolled atrial fibrillation.

There are certain factors that may overestimate (any LVOT obstruction, systemic hypertension, premature beats, catheter entrapped in mitral subvalvular apparatus, catheter placed too close to the mitral valve) or underestimate (inappropriate catheter and/or contrast volume used, slow injection, severely dilated left ventricular cavity, catheter placed too distally) the severity of mitral regurgitation (Figure 9.3). Hence, the operator must take these factors into consideration when making a final conclusion on the grade of mitral regurgitation. On the other hand, for patients with a smaller ventricle or with decreased cardiac output, less volume (30 mL) and a lower rate (10–12 mL/second) should be used for qualitative assessment of LV systolic function and segmental wall motion on biplane views (Table 9.3).

Quantitative assessment of the LV function can be done by calculating ejection fraction from measured LV end-diastolic and-end systolic volumes [LVEF = (LVEDV – LVESV)/LVEDV]. In patients where the amount of contrast is an issue, biplane left

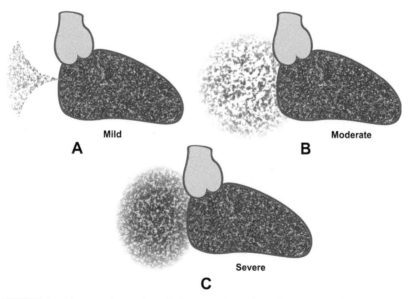

Mild

A

Moderate

B

Severe

C

FIGURE 9.3 Diagram of RAO view of left ventriculography in the presence of mitral regurgitation shows mild (**Panel A**), moderate (**Panel B**), and severe (**Panel C**) mitral regurgitation.

TABLE 9.3   Angiographic classification of left ventricular segmental wall motion.

LAO 50- to 60-degree view – Basal septal, anterolateral, and posterolateral walls
RAO 30- to 40-degree view – Anterobasal, anterolateral, apical, inferoapical, and inferobasal walls
- Normal
- Hypokinetic – Decreased systolic inward motion
- Akinetic – Absence of systolic inward motion
- Dyskinetic – Paradoxical systolic outward motion

TABLE 9.4   Optimal angiographic views in certain pathologies.

- Muscular VSD – LAO 60-degree view with 25-degree cranial angulation
- Membranous VSD – LAO 80-degree view
- RV Infundibulum – RAO 30-degree view with 40-degree cranial angulation
- Prosthetic Mitral Valve – RAO with or without angulation
- Prosthetic Aortic Valve – LAO with or without angulation

ventriculography with a multipurpose catheter with hand injection of 8–10 mL of contrast is recommended, as described in Chapter 7.

It is generally accepted that for certain cardiac problems, certain angiographic views are recommended (Table 9.4).

After all the appropriate images are obtained, the syringe is reattached to the manifold. The pigtail catheter is flushed with heparinized saline, and LV systolic and end-diastolic pressures are measured and recorded on 200 mm Hg pressure and 50 mm/second speed scales, accordingly. The catheter is subsequently withdrawn into the ascending aorta where arterial pressure is recorded and the presence or absence of a trans-aortic valve gradient is determined. Upon completion of the pressure recording, the pigtail catheter is withdrawn below the aortic arch into the descending aorta.

JUDKINS RIGHT CATHETER

The JR end-hole catheter can be used for crossing the aortic valve. The catheter is advanced in 60-degree LAO projection from the sinotubular junction until its tip buckles in the coronary cusp. This is followed by slight withdrawal with a slight clockwise rotation applied to the catheter while the patient is asked to take a deep breath. With this maneuver, the catheter tip usually prolapses into the LV cavity, where it is stabilized in the mid-ventricular position co-axial with the longitudinal axis of the LV in RAO 30-degree projection.

If an atypical anatomic configuration or sclero-calcific changes of the aortic valve impede the process of crossing the valve with the described method, the guidewire support technique can be used to achieve the goal. The catheter slides over the 0.035-inch, J-tip guidewire until the tip of the wire gets covered by the tip of the catheter. The guidewire stays inside the catheter while the catheter is rotated in the ascending aorta in 60-degree LAO projection. The catheter is advanced until its tip buckles in the coronary cusp, followed by a slight withdrawal with a simultaneous clockwise half-turn. This turn can be accompanied by slight in-and-out motion of the catheter in order to transmit the applied torque. As the catheter tip straightens from being buckled in the cusp, it prolapses into the ventricular cavity, where it gets stabilized in the mid-ventricular position coaxial with the longitudinal axis of the left ventricle. The other method utilizes the guidewire, but this time the guidewire leads the catheter into the left ventricular cavity. The catheter slides over the 0.035-inch, J-tip guidewire (0.035-inch, soft, straight-tip guidewire is preferred) until the tip of the guidewire gets covered by the tip of the catheter. The guidewire stays inside the catheter while the catheter is rotated in the ascending aorta just above the aortic sinuses in 30-degree RAO and 60-degree LAO projections. At this point the guidewire is advanced against the valve. Sometimes the guidewire slips straight across the valve, but if not the operator gently pushes it forward, with the catheter following, until 3–4 cm of the guidewire's distal tip is buckled and curled back in the aortic sinus. Then the catheter is withdrawn slightly followed by gentle withdrawal of the wire. When the curve of the wire straightens, it usually prolapses through the valve. The operator slides the catheter over the wire into the left ventricle. If and when ventriculography is required, the JR catheter should be exchanged over the long (240 cm) J-tip, 0.035-inch guidewire for an angled pigtail catheter, since it is not recommended to perform left ventriculography using end-hole catheters due to increased risk of endocardial staining or damage. In order to accomplish this exchange, the operator disconnects the JR4 catheter from the manifold and passes through it the long exchange wire until the wire tip appears in the LV cavity. The wire is fixed in position and the catheter is withdrawn over the wire. The angled pigtail catheter is placed over the guidewire and slides into the LV. The key point of an exchange maneuver is to preserve the position of the wire tip in the LV cavity, which can be monitored by fluoroscopy. Once the angled pigtail catheter is in position, the guidewire is withdrawn.

AMPLATZ LEFT CATHETER

The end hole AL catheter can be used for crossing the stenotic aortic valve (especially in patients with a dilated ascending aorta). In order to cross the aortic valve, the operator advances the catheter over the 0.035-inch long exchange straight soft-tip guidewire through the arterial sheath into the aorta under fluoroscopic guidance. The guidewire stays inside the catheter while the catheter is rotated in the ascending aorta above the aortic sinuses in 30-degree RAO projection. At this point, the guidewire is advanced towards the valve. Sometimes the guidewire slips straight across the valve; on these occasions, the operator reorients the tip of the catheter towards the high velocity jet of aortic stenosis, which can be monitored when the wire and the tip of the catheter are moved by it. Severe calcification may outline the valve and slight movement of the calcified tips of the leaflet can be visible during fluoroscopy assisting the operator to direct the wire towards it. When the tip of the wire prolapses through the valve into the ventricle, the wire gets fixed and the AL catheter slides over it into the LV cavity. The wire is removed and LV pressure is recorded. Subsequently, the AL catheter can be exchanged over the long exchange wire to an angled pigtail catheter.

Radiologic Anatomy of the Heart and Right Ventriculography

As mentioned previously, knowledge of cardiac structures projected in different angiographic views is of utmost importance. Right heart structures outlined in different projects are illustrated in Figure 9.4.

Right ventriculography is performed rarely by invasive cardiologists in the contemporary adult cardiac catheterization laboratory, mainly because 3D echocardiography and MRI provide more accurate information for clinical decision making. Right ventriculography is a relatively safe procedure unless done in patients with severe pulmonary hypertension. In such patients, it can be done with a reduced contrast volume, which is usually injected with a straight-body pigtail catheter or Berman balloon-directed, multisided-hole, closed-end catheter (see Chapter 3, Figure 3.7). It is very important to measure right-sided pressures before proceeding with right ventriculography. The technique for placing a Berman catheter into the right ventricle (RV) is similar to a routine Swan-Ganz balloon-tipped

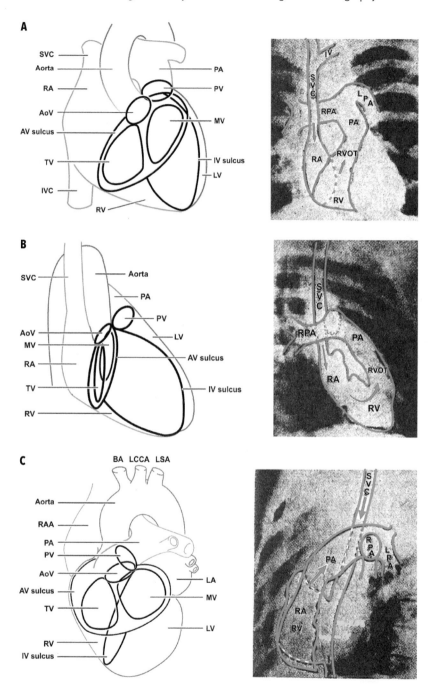

FIGURE 9.4   Radiologic anatomy of the right heart, pulmonary arteries, and caval veins is shown with corresponding cardiac diagrams. **Panel A**: PA view; **Panel B**: RAO view; **Panel C**: LAO view; **Panel D**: LL view.

D

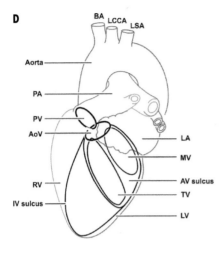
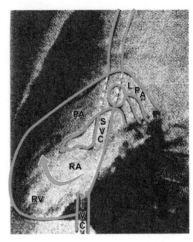

FIGURE 9.4   (*Continued*)

catheter placement. In regards to standard, straight-body pigtail catheter, the operator can use a tip deflector or bent-wire to direct the catheter to the RV, but usually an exchange-wire technique will be used after accessing the RV with the Swan-Ganz catheter. Biplane ventriculography should be performed in PA and LAO views both with slight 15- to 20-degree cranial angulation to reduce foreshortening of the RV cavity and improve separation of the RV outflow tract from the pulmonary artery. After RV pressure is recorded the operator proceeds with preparations to perform ventriculography. Typical settings are 25–50 mL contrast volume injected at a rate of 15–25 mL/second. A frame rate set at 15 frames/sec is used in order to assess RV volumes and calculate RV ejection fraction.

Aortography

Aortography is performed to assess severity of aortic valve regurgitation (Table 9.5; Figure 9.5), to define aortic anatomy (presence

TABLE 9.5   **Angiographic classification of aortic regurgitation severity.**

1. Mild (1+) – Minimal and incomplete opacification of the LV, which clears with each cardiac cycle.
2. Moderate (2+) – Complete but faint opacification of the LV after several cardiac cycles.
3. Moderate to Severe (3+) – Complete opacification of the LV after more than one cardiac cycle with the same intensity as aorta.
4. Severe (4+) – Complete and very intense opacification of the LV within one cardiac cycle.

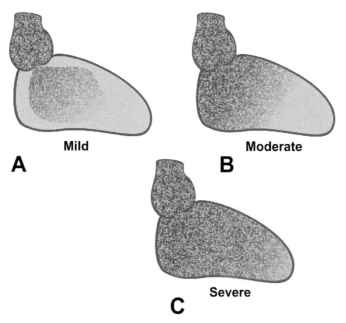

FIGURE 9.5   Diagram shows left ventriculography in RAO view and in presence of **(Panel A)** mild, **(Panel B)** moderate, and **(Panel C)** severe aortic regurgitation.

and site of coarctation, location and size of an aneurysm and dissection), to detect aortic arch type, and to locate anomalous coronary arteries and bypass grafts.

There are certain factors that the operator must take into consideration when making the final conclusion on grading of aortic regurgitation. The following factors may overestimate (systemic hypertension, catheter placed too close to the aortic valve) or underestimate (inappropriate catheter type and/or contrast volume used, slow injection, severely dilated aortic root, catheter placed too proximally) the severity of aortic regurgitation. When initiating the procedure, the operator places the straight 6-Fr pigtail catheter over the 0.035-inch, J-tip guidewire above the sinotubular junction in 60-degree LAO projection. Then the wire is removed and aortic pressure is recorded. It is important to determine the location of the catheter tip by doing test injections, in order to exclude the possibility of the catheter being placed in the false lumen in patients with aortic dissection.

The usual settings of the power injector for aortography are 40–60 mL of dye with an injection rate of 15–20 mL/sec. Angiography in 60-degree LAO with 10- to 20-degree cranial angulation and 30-degree RAO projections is then initiated and aortography performed. The slight cranial angulation is added in an attempt to better visualize aortic root and arch and to decrease overlap between the ascending and descending aortic segments. Angiography should continue until the contrast is cleared. Arch aortography in LAO 40-degree view is performed with the patient's head turned and extended to the right.

If aortography shows aortic coarctation, a pressure gradient should be measured while slowly withdrawing the catheter under continuous pressure monitoring. In general a pressure gradient ≥ 50 mm Hg requires correction.

Aortography of the descending and abdominal aorta can be performed utilizing the straight PA and left lateral projections. Aortography of the descending aorta is performed with a straight pigtail catheter positioned distal to the left subclavian artery, and abdominal aortography is performed with the tip of the straight pigtail catheter positioned at the T12 vertebra level. The benefit of using these views are (1) evaluation of the abdominal aorta in two orthogonal views, (2) better visualization of the ostia of the mesenteric vessels in left lateral view, and (3) ostia of renal arteries in the PA view, which can be useful if selective angiography of those vessels is considered. Angiography of the aortic bifurcation and iliac arteries can be done with the straight pigtail catheter in PA view, occasionally combined with 30- to 45-degree RAO or LAO views if a biplane system is used.

Pulmonary Artery Angiography

Pulmonary artery angiography is a relatively safe procedure unless done in patients with severe pulmonary hypertension. In such patients it is usually not recommended, but can be done with reduced volumes of contrast injected through a straight pigtail, Berman balloon-directed multi-hole (see Chapter 3, Figure 3.7), or Grollman catheter (see Chapter 3, Figure 3.8). The Grollman catheter, with its preformed shape and ring-up pigtail, allows for easy passage into the RV. Using clockwise rotation with simultaneous advancement places the tip of the catheter into the RV outflow tract from where the J-tip guidewire can be navigated through the pulmonic valve into the main pulmonary artery (Figure 9.6).

It is strongly recommended to measure right-sided pressures and oxygen saturations before proceeding with pulmonary

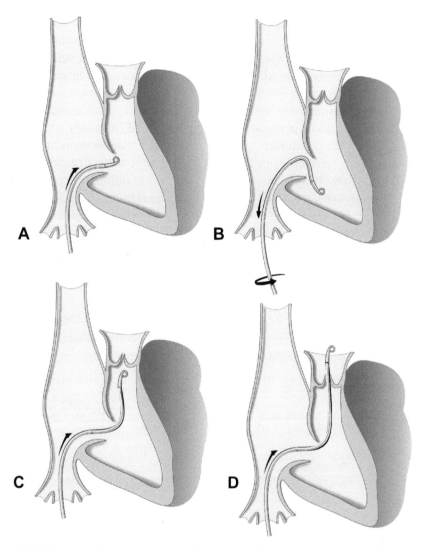

FIGURE 9.6   The following steps are used in accessing the pulmonary artery with the Grollman catheter: After the initial advance into the RV (**Panel A**), a clockwise rotation with simultaneous advancement places the tip of the catheter into the RV outflow tract (**Panel B**); the catheter is navigated toward the pulmonic valve (**Panel C**) and from there into the main pulmonary artery (**Panel D**).

angiography. In regards to the standard straight pigtail catheter, the operator can use a tip deflector or bent-wire to direct it to the pulmonary artery, but usually the exchange wire technique will be used after accessing the main pulmonary artery with a Swan-Ganz catheter. After pulmonary pressures are recorded, the operator proceeds with preparation to perform pulmonary angiography (see the earlier discussion of aortography technique). Biplane pulmonary angiography is performed for the main pulmonary artery and its bifurcation in straight AP view with 30-degree cranial angulation, in LAO 45-degree view for the left pulmonary artery, and RAO 45-degree view for the right pulmonary artery. Typical settings are 30–50 mL of contrast volume injected at a rate of 15–20 mL/second. The higher the pulmonary pressure, the lower the volume and rate of injection must be in order to avoid acute elevation of pressure potentially resulting in acute right-sided heart failure. When all the above steps are completed and right heart pressures rechecked, the catheter is removed over the wire through the venous sheath. When crossing valves or performing left or right ventriculography, aortography, or pulmonary angiography, the operator should be well aware of the major complications associated with the procedure, and how to handle these effectively.

WHAT IF AN OPERATOR ENCOUNTERS ONE OF THE FOLLOWING PROBLEMS?

Acute Valvular Damage

Acute valvular damage occurs rarely, unless the operator is dealing with a calcified aortic bioprothesis, which can be damaged while attempting to cross it. It is recommended to use a soft, straight-tip, 0.035-inch guidewire to cross this type of valve, and then over the wire deploy the catheter. A normal aortic valve is pretty resistant to damage, unless the operator is inexperienced and overaggressive while trying to cross it. Mitral valve–supporting apparatus can be damaged during left ventriculography when a power injector is used. This can occur if the pigtail catheter is entangled in the mitral valve chordal apparatus. Severe, acute mitral regurgitation can result with dramatic clinical deterioration.

Ventricular Perforation or Rupture

Ventricular perforation or rupture can rarely occur as a result of overly aggressive manipulation of the guidewire or catheter inside the ventricular cavity. The other potential cause is injection of contrast into the ventricular cavity when the catheter is placed against the wall. This, in mild cases, may lead to endocardial staining with accompanied ventricular arrhythmias and, in the worst-case scenario, lead to rupture of the ventricular wall with catastrophic consequences for the patient. During contrast injection, the operator should be ready to withdraw the catheter immediately if myocardial staining or ventricular tachycardia occurs.

Complete Heart Block

Complete heart block may occur in patients with baseline right bundle branch block. In general, the block occurs due to transient damage of the left bundle branch during placement of the pigtail catheter into the LV cavity, although it can also happen with any other type of catheter.

Aortic Dissection

Dissection of the ascending aorta or arch is an indication for surgical repair, although in some cases intra-aortic stenting can be performed. In most cases of descending or abdominal aortic dissections that are not complicated by involving vital organs and are clinically asymptomatic, close monitoring and conservative management is sufficient. Retrograde aortic dissection is mostly caused by overly aggressive manipulation of the catheter or guidewire and can be prevented by using a cautious approach. The vast majority of these dissections are self-contained and self-healed and do not require surgical or percutaneous intervention to seal them. Aortography in the presence of an existing aortic dissection can lead to propagation of the dissection if the catheter is accidentally placed in the false lumen and is accompanied by power injection. The operator always needs to make sure that the catheter tip is not placed in the false lumen by checking the aortic pressure waveforms and aspirating blood from the distal tip of the catheter without any problems. Proximal aortic dissections can extend distally along the left posterior lateral surface of the aorta and into the left iliac artery. The false lumen is commonly entered in such cases if arterial access is obtained via the left common femoral artery approach. The true lumen is usually entered either from the right radial/brachial or right femoral approach. When considering aortography, a test injection should be done first to make sure that the catheter tip is in the true lumen. If the test injection shows delayed washout or swirling of contrast, it should be assumed that the catheter is in the false lumen.

Aortic Rupture

Aortic rupture is extremely rare, and will require emergency cardiothoracic or vascular surgery intervention. Occasionally, it can be managed by placement of covered intraaortic stents by vascular surgery.

Small and Horizontally Positioned LV

In these cases, straight rather than angled pigtail catheters are preferred because of greater flexibility. In patients with smaller ventricles, where nonarrhythmogenic positioning of an angled pigtail catheter is difficult, a straight pigtail catheter can be used, since they are easily rotated inside the LV.

For other potential complications, such as myocardial infarction, stroke, pulmonary edema, vasovagal reaction, ventricular arrhythmias, peripheral thromboembolism, and air embolism, see Chapter 6.

References

1. Gigliotti OS, Babb JD, Dieter RS, et al. Optimal use of left ventriculography at the time of cardiac catheterization: A consensus statement from the society for cardiovascular angiography and interventions. *Catheter Cardiovasc Interv.* 2015;85(2):181-191.

2. Casserly IP, Messenger JC. Technique and catheters. *Cardiol Clin.* 2009; 27:417-432.

CHAPTER 10

Right Heart Catheterization

"The best way out of difficulty is through it."

—Anonymous

Indications and Contraindications of the Procedure

Every procedure performed in the cardiac catheterization laboratory has its own indications and contraindications. The same can be said about right heart catheterization (Tables 10.1 and 10.2). The majority of right heart catheterization procedures are done with a multilumen, 7- to 8-Fr, balloon-tipped flotation catheter with thermodilution cardiac output measurement capabilities.[1,2] Prior to insertion, the operator checks the balloon for the presence of an air leak by inflating it under water, flushes the lumen of the catheter, zeroes the pressure transducer at the level of the mid right atrium, and ensures that no air bubbles are present in the tubing or in the catheter after its distal port is connected to the pressure transducer (to avoid "underdamped" or "overdamped" pressure tracings). Recorded pressure will be too low if a transducer is positioned too high and vice versa; for every inch that the heart is away from the reference point of the transducer, a 2 mm Hg degree of error will be introduced.

If left bundle branch block is present on the ECG, the right heart catheterization procedure should be done with extreme caution in order to avoid iatrogenic right bundle branch block that could result in complete heart block. It is recommended to have a temporary pacemaker ready in case a prolonged episode of iatrogenic complete

TABLE 10.1   Indications for diagnostic right heart catheterization.

INDICATION	NOTES
Acute myocardial infarction	Complicated by hypotension, HF, sinus tachycardia, RV infarction, or mechanical complications (VSD, tamponade, or acute MR)
Assessment of volume status	When physical examination is unreliable
Severe left ventricular failure	To guide inotropic, diuretic, and afterload reduction management
Differentiation between various shock states	Cardiogenic, distributive, or hypovolemic; and guidance for therapies
Risk stratification for patients during heart transplant evaluation	
Cardiac tamponade	Although Echo is the diagnostic test of choice, PA cath may be used when Echo is not readily available or Echo findings are not diagnostic and risk or difficulty of pericardiocentesis is high.
Assessment of level and magnitude of intracardiac shunt	Especially if TTE is nondiagnostic
Differentiation between constrictive and restrictive cardiac physiology	
Severe pulmonary hypertension	

TABLE 10.2   Contraindications to diagnostic right heart catheterization.

ABSOLUTE	RELATIVE
Right-sided endocarditis	Coagulopathy (INR > 2, platelets < $20 \times 10^3/mm^3$)
Mechanical tricuspid or pulmonic valve	Bioprosthetic tricuspid or pulmonic valve
Thrombus or tumor in right heart chamber	Newly implanted pacemaker or defibrillator (unless fluoroscopic guidance is used)
Terminal illness for which aggressive management is futile	LBBB (temporary pacing should be available)

heart block develops. After all appropriate preprocedure preparations are completed, the operator advances the tip of the catheter through the 7- to 8-Fr venous sheath up to the 20-cm mark on the catheter prior to inflating the balloon. This ensures that the tip of the catheter passes the tip of the sheath. It is extremely important to refrain from advancing the catheter if resistance is noted due to the risk of vessel perforation. After the balloon is inflated successfully and pressure is recorded, the operator advances the catheter antegrade toward the right heart under fluoroscopic guidance.

Femoral Vein Approach

When utilizing the femoral vein approach, the catheter is advanced through the inferior vena cava (IVC) towards the right atrium (RA) and subsequently into the superior vena cava (SVC) (Figure 10.1). While navigating the catheter through the IVC with the inflated balloon, deviation of the catheter tip from its paraspinal position may suggest entry into a branch vein (hepatic, renal).

To correct this error, the operator withdraws the catheter, torques it slightly, and then advances it. In order to place the catheter into the SVC, the operator slowly torques the catheter counterclockwise in PA view and directs the tip to the lateral wall of the RA

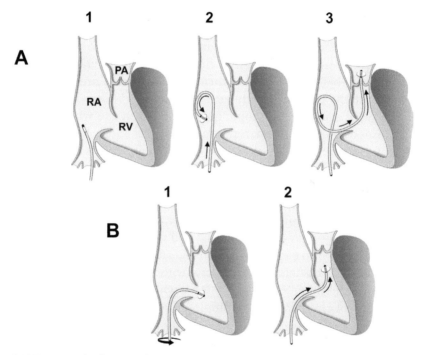

FIGURE 10.1   The drawings show two approaches to accessing the pulmonary artery with a Swan-Ganz catheter via the femoral approach. **Panel A**: While in the RA, the Swan-Ganz catheter is torqued to direct the tip towards the lateral wall of the RA and is advanced until the tip touches the atrial wall. Further advancement of the catheter builds a loop that points its tip t towards the tricuspid valve, The catheter passes through the valve into the RV and PA upon further advancement. **Panel B**: The catheter tip is turned toward the patient's left side by clockwise torque, positioned in the lower part of the RA towards its anteromedial wall, and advanced across the tricuspid valve into the RV. Next the catheter is torqued clockwise so that the tip turns cranially towards the RVOT.

(Figure 10.1A). Subsequent additional counterclockwise rotation and gentle advancement usually allows passage of the catheter tip into the SVC, which is contiguous with the posterolateral wall of the RA. These slow, step-by-step, counterclockwise (half-turn) rotations should be done using the fingers of both hands, with the right hand on catheter hub adaptor, and the left hand assisting in turning of the catheter near the end of the venous sheath. After each turn, a small amount of time is allowed for transmission of the torque that is applied at the base of the catheter. This step-wise rotation allows the operator to avoid catheter over-torqueing and kinking. To facilitate this process, minimal "in-and-out" movement of the catheter is performed. If this maneuver turns out to be unsuccessful, the operator disconnects the proximal end of the right heart catheter from the manifold and advances the J-tip, 0.025-inch guidewire through the catheter under fluoroscopic guidance. The operator places a 3-way stopcock on the proximal end of the guidewire and locks it to allow for easier torque of the wire, if needed, and to prevent the guidewire from being lost. After this is done, the operator slightly deflates the balloon and, while turning the catheter, probes for the ostium of the SVC by gently advancing and withdrawing the tip of the wire under fluoroscopic guidance. When the wire is safely positioned in the SVC, the right heart catheter slides over it and is placed near the junction of the innominate vein. This is followed by removal of the wire, with subsequent aspiration and flushing of the catheter, and SVC pressure recording.

Next, the operator aspirates from the distal port of the right heart catheter 1–2 mL blood, then sequentially attaches three 5-mL heparinized syringes to the manifold and aspirates 1–2 mL of blood from the SVC into each of those syringes to measure mean oxygen saturation. The catheter is flushed and withdrawn towards the lower SVC (near the junction with the RA), where the above-described procedure of obtaining blood samples for oximetry is repeated. The catheter is again flushed well and withdrawn into the RA, where the pressure tracings are recorded and 3 samples of blood are obtained in 3 positions (high, mid, and low RA), in the same way it was done for the SVC. The catheter is thoroughly flushed after each step.

Next, the balloon is inflated and the catheter tip is turned toward the patient's left side by clockwise torque, positioned in the lower part of the RA towards its anteromedial wall, and advanced across the tricuspid valve into the RV, where pressure is recorded and 3 oximetry samples are obtained. If a shunt is suspected 3 samples of blood are obtained in 3 positions: mid RV, RV apex, and RV outflow tract (RVOT). Occasionally, the advancement of the catheter into the RV is met with difficulty. Three alternative approaches can be taken: First, the catheter is placed in the lower IVC, and then slow, clockwise torque is applied until the catheter tip is pointed to the right side of the patient's body. When this is accomplished, the catheter with the inflated balloon is slowly advanced towards the hepatic vein. As it is placed in the hepatic vein, the operator advances the catheter gently, shaping the catheter curve. The catheter is brought back into the IVC and is advanced into the RA, where the steeper curve facilitates its advancement into the RV (Figure 10.1B). Second, while in the RA, the balloon is deflated, the catheter is gently torqued to direct the tip towards the lateral wall of the RA (approximately 9 to 11 o'clock on the screen), and is advanced gently until the tip touches the atrial wall. Further gentle, forward pressure applied to the catheter against the atrial wall causes a loop to form. Once the loop is formed, the balloon is inflated, causing the tip to point toward the tricuspid valve, so that with further pushing the tip passes through the tricuspid valve into the RV (Figure 10.1A). The third option is a combination of the first and second approaches with advancement of a 0.025-inch, J-tip guidewire. When the guidewire safely crosses the tricuspid valve and enters the RV, the catheter slides slowly over into the RV, the wire is removed, and the balloon is inflated.

Occasionally, some operators inject 1.5 mL normal saline or a half-and-half mixture of normal saline with contrast dye into the balloon, to allow gravity to help the balloon to cross through the tricuspid valve. When successful, the fluid is aspirated and the balloon reinflated with air. With the second approach, the process of advancing the catheter into the RVOT and into the main PA is simple, since this route corresponds to the natural curve of the catheter. Other approaches require some dexterity from the operator. In order to place the right heart catheter into the PA with the first approach, the catheter is positioned in the body of the RV away from its apex. The operator torques the catheter clockwise under fluoroscopic guidance. This clockwise rotation should be done by the operator using the fingers of both hands, with the right hand on the catheter hub adaptor, and the left hand assisting in turning the catheter near the end of the venous sheath. This maneuver is frequently accompanied by enlargement of the loop. Applying gentle back-traction takes the large curve off and maintains the same curve size. At a certain point, the catheter tip turns upward toward the RVOT. When this occurs, the operator should quickly advance the catheter into the PA. Advancement may be facilitated with the patient taking a deep breath, which augments pulmonary flow. In difficult cases, placing a 0.025-inch, J-tip guidewire to stiffen the catheter may facilitate its advancement into the PA. Occasionally, the catheter tip is placed in the RVOT, but advancement of an inflated balloon tipped catheter is not possible. In this case, a 0.025-inch, J-tip guidewire is run through the tip of the catheter towards the pulmonary valve. When the valve is successfully crossed, the balloon is deflated and the tip of the catheter slides gently over the wire into the main PA. The wire is then removed, and the balloon is inflated. Once in the left or right PA, the pressure tracing is recorded and oximetry samples are obtained. Then the catheter tip is advanced into the "wedge" position (occasionally asking the patient to take a deep breath or cough to facilitate positioning the tip of the catheter in the "wedge" position), where the PA occlusive pressure is recorded at the end of expiration. In cases where wedging the tip of the catheter is difficult, the operator releases a small amount (0.5 mL) of air from the balloon to decrease its size and slowly advances the catheter to facilitate wedging. The "wedge" pressure should be monitored carefully, to avoid "overwedging" since the likelihood of vessel rupture and infarction is directly proportional to the catheter being overwedged. The operator should avoid vigorous flushing of the catheter when in "wedge" position in order to prevent rupture of the vessel. If the operator is unsure of the correct "wedge" position, an oximetry sample should be obtained and measured to prove the true "wedge" position of the catheter tip (arterial O_2 saturation). Other signs of optimal wedge position include a stationary tip position, characteristic waveforms, and mean wedge pressure less than mean PA pressure.

When "wedge" pressure is obtained, the catheter tip is moved back to the main PA and an attempt is made to advance it with the inflated balloon towards the opposite branch (usually right) of the PA. If the maneuver meets with difficulty, the operator uses a 0.025-inch wire to navigate the catheter toward the appropriate main branch. When the distal tip of the catheter is safely placed, the balloon is deflated, pressure is recorded, and oximetry samples are obtained. After this step, the catheter is flushed, withdrawn, and repositioned in the main PA, where oximetry samples are obtained and thermodilution cardiac output is measured. Simultaneously, the arterial sheath is flushed and 3 oximetry samples are obtained in order to calculate cardiac output with the Fick method (see Chapter 19).

It is important to record all pressures at end expiration if the patient is able to hold his/her breath without involuntarily performing Valsalva maneuver, since the effect of intrathoracic pressure on intracardiac pressures is minimal under physiological conditions at end expiration.

Right Internal Jugular Vein Approach

When utilizing the right internal jugular (RIJ) vein approach for right heart catheterization, the catheter is advanced through the sheath towards the SVC, the balloon is inflated, and the vena caval pressure recorded (Figure 10.2).

The steps for obtaining blood for oximetry have been described earlier in this chapter. Placing the right heart catheter into the PA through the RIJ approach is relatively easy, since this approach will provide a route that corresponds to the natural curve of the catheter such that the catheter tip faces toward the RVOT and the operator can advance the catheter into the PA. In order to place the catheter into the IVC from the RA, the operator inflates the balloon and slowly, under fluoroscopic guidance, torques the catheter clockwise to point the catheter tip towards the right side of the patient's body and the lateral wall of the RA. If this maneuver for cannulating the IVC turns out to be unsuccessful, the operator advances the 0.025-inch, J-tip guidewire through the catheter under fluoroscopic guidance, and, while turning the catheter, probes for the ostium of the IVC by gently advancing and withdrawing the tip of the wire. When the wire is positioned in the lower IVC (at the level of L4–L5 vertebrae) the right heart catheter slides over the wire. This

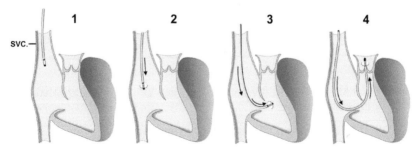

FIGURE 10.2 The drawing illustrates the steps used in accessing the pulmonary artery with a Swan-Ganz catheter from the internal jugular, subclavian, or basilic vein approach.

is followed by removal of the wire, aspiration and flushing of the catheter, deflation of the balloon, recording of the IVC pressure, and obtaining oximetry samples.

The methods described for the RIJ approach are used in two other techniques: The subclavian vein approach and the basilic vein approach (for access techniques for both veins, see Chapter 5) are discussed briefly below.

SUBCLAVIAN VEIN APPROACH

After the Swan-Ganz catheter is advanced through the sheath, the balloon is inflated and moved towards the SVC. From this point on, the approach is similar to the RIJ technique as described above.

BASILIC VEIN APPROACH

After the Swan-Ganz catheter is advanced over the J-tip guide-wire through the sheath towards the axillary vein and subsequently through the subclavian vein, the balloon is inflated and moved towards the SVC. From this point on, the approach is similar to the RIJ technique described above.

Cannulation of the Coronary Sinus

When approaching the coronary sinus from the RIJ, the catheter tip entering the RA is initially pointed to the lateral wall (right side of the patient in AP view). The catheter is subsequently torqued counterclockwise and moved forward to just enter the right ventricle. At this point additional slight counterclockwise torque is applied and the catheter is slowly pushed back until right ventricular pressure changes to right atrial pressure. When this occurs the operator gently advances the catheter which in general cannulates the coronary sinus located posteriorly to the tricuspid annulus.

WHAT IF AN OPERATOR ENCOUNTERS ONE OF THE FOLLOWING PROBLEMS?

Inability to Advance the Catheter Within the Sheath

After successfully obtaining venous access and placing the sheath there is a problem of advancing the Swan-Ganz catheter within the sheath. The most likely cause is sheath kinking. (Please see steps for management of a similar problem in Chapter 5).

Difficulty Inflating the Balloon

After successfully obtaining venous access and advancing the Swan-Ganz catheter within the sheath, the operator may have difficulty inflating the balloon. The most obvious cause is that the tip of the catheter did not pass the tip of the sheath yet. A simple solution is to gently advance the catheter under fluoroscopy and reinflate the balloon slowly. If the problem remains, the operator should deflate the balloon, remove the catheter, and check the balloon for leaks by inflating it under water. If there is no problem with the balloon, reattempt placing the catheter. If the same problem occurs again, aspirate and flush the venous sheath, and under fluoroscopy inject several mL of contrast dye, in order to be able to visualize the problem and make a decision based on the obtained image.

Resistance in Advancing the Catheter After Balloon Inflation

After successfully obtaining venous access and advancing the Swan-Ganz catheter within the sheath, the operator inflates the balloon and continues advancing the Swan-Ganz catheter in the central vein towards the right atrium. If the catheter suddenly meets resistance, the operator should stop; *do not advance the catheter against resistance.* Rather, withdraw the catheter, torque it clockwise or counter-clockwise, and attempt to advance the catheter again. This maneuver helps to avoid a venous branch, which could be the cause of resistance if the balloon-tipped catheter accidently migrated into it. If resistance persists, the tip of the catheter should be moved slightly back from the point of resistance, the catheter flushed, and several mL of contrast dye injected under fluoroscopy. This allows the operator to visualize the problem and make a decision based on the obtained image. If dealing with a complete occlusion or a fragile intravascular mass obstructing the vessel, this vascular route needs to be abandoned.

Arrhythmias

As a balloon-tipped catheter enters the RA and passes to the RV, the primary complications are arrhythmias which in most cases are minor in nature and temporary in character. These are caused by the physical contact of the balloon-tipped catheter with the RV endocardium and can be easily terminated, either by slight withdrawal of the catheter or by quick advancement of the catheter into the PA. Sustained atrial or ventricular arrhythmias requiring treatment occur primarily in patients with myocardial ischemia, myocardial infarction, or preexisting atrial or ventricular arrhythmias.

When these occur, the operator and cath lab personnel should follow the current ACLS guidelines. In the presence of LBBB, iatrogenic RBBB by right heart catheterization results in complete heart block, so it is very important for cath lab personnel to have a temporary transvenous pacemaker ready to be inserted. If for some reason a delay occurs, and there is inadequate or absent escape rhythm, transcutaneous pacing should be initiated. Meanwhile, asking the patient to cough and rhythmically touching the RV endocardium with the tip of the Swan-Ganz catheter causes mechanically induced ventricular depolarization and supports circulation until a steady heart rhythm can be restored.

Vasovagal Reaction

A prolonged episode of bradycardia accompanied by hypotension, nausea, and diaphoresis can be a manifestation of a vasovagal reaction, especially in anxious patients with volume depletion. This generally benign complication responds to rapid volume administration combined with 0.5–1.0 mg intravenous atropine and elevation of the lower extremities. On rare occasions, intravenous pressors are required.

Existing Pacemaker or ICD Devices

In cases where a recently placed temporary or permanent pacemaker or implantable cardioverter-defibrillator are present, the RIJ approach is recommended when placing a Swan-Ganz catheter under fluoroscopy in order to minimize maneuvering and torqueing of the catheter, and to decrease the chance of dislodgement of the leads.

Unintended Cannulation of the Coronary Sinus

Accidental cannulation of the coronary sinus can be recognized by the appearance of the catheter going into the right ventricle on the fluoroscopy image, but with atrial pressure tracings. Another hint is the absence of ventricular ectopy when the catheter shape looks as if it is directed towards the RVOT. A definite answer can be provided by a test injection. If the injection shows the catheter to be in the coronary sinus, the catheter should be pulled back, unless a selective coronary sinus venogram is required.

Atrial or Ventricular Perforation

RA or RV perforation during right heart catheterization under flu-oroscopy guidance is extremely rare. This devastating complication is frequently preceded by pain and may be accompanied by vasova-gal symptoms when blood enters the pericardium. These symptoms are followed by the development of cardiac tamponade with hemo-dynamic compromise, requiring, in the worst-case scenario, emer-gent pericardiocentesis. The cardiothoracic surgery team should be notified if a patient's hemodynamic status continues to deteriorate and pericardiocentesis is unsuccessful.

If the patient was anticoagulated prior to cardiac catheteriza-tion, an attempt should be made to reverse anticoagulation. It is recommended to try to remove most of the free blood from the pericardial space before reversing systemic heparinization with pro-tamine, since early administration of protamine may cause trans-formation of the pericardial free blood into a gel-type fluid that can potentially make the process of aspiration through the pericardio-centesis catheter virtually impossible.

Pressure Damping

When attempting to place the Swan-Ganz catheter into the main pulmonary artery from the femoral approach, the operator fre-quently does a lot of clockwise torqueing of the catheter. During this process the pressure tracing should be watched carefully, since damping of the pressure, which may go unnoticed by the operator who is preoccupied with catheter maneuvering, is an early sign of catheter kinking. Kinking should be avoided, since a complex kink is hard to manage (see Chapter 5). Other potential causes of the damped pressure include placing the tip of the catheter against the vessel wall, a thrombus in the lumen of the catheter, air in the stop-cocks or pressure transducer, and a faulty transducer.

Pulmonary Artery Branch Rupture

Rupture of small branches of the pulmonary artery occur mostly when an operator does not notice that the tip of the Swan-Ganz catheter has migrated distally into the vessel and inflates the bal-loon quickly (rarely happens in the cardiac catheterization labora-tory), or when a stiff, end-hole catheter was used to aggressively obtain true wedge pressure. The clinical presentation of this com-plication is dramatic, with sudden onset of cough with hemoptysis followed by cardiovascular collapse. If this happens, the operator should not deflate the balloon, but should immediately turn the patient on the side of the affected lung and call cardiothoracic surgery while attempting to medically stabilize the patient. The other potential complication of a wedged catheter is ischemia/infarction of the lung, but this complication is, fortunately, extremely rare.

Wedging Problems

When the pressure tracing shows a continuous rise of a pressure when the catheter tip is in wedge position, it signals a phenomenon called "overwedging," which is most often encountered during balloon inflation when the catheter tip is located too far distally in the pulmonary vasculature. "Overwedging" places the patient under imminent risk for pulmonary artery rupture. The operator should realize this immediately, deflate the balloon, and withdraw the catheter.

In contrast, when mean wedge pressure is higher than mean pulmonary artery pressure, it may suggest that the Swan-Ganz catheter tip is not wedged in lung zone III (usually the most dependent portions of the lungs). The operator should deflate the balloon, withdraw the catheter, re-inflate the balloon, and reposition the distal tip of the catheter.

Catheter "Whip" or "Ringing"

Another common phenomenon occurring with right heart catheterization is "catheter whip," or "ringing," which in most cases is due to the vigorous motion of the balloon-tipped catheter in PA or RV when pressure is recorded. This can be reduced by repositioning the catheter, or by filling the catheter with one-to-one saline contrast mixture.

References

1. Mueller HS, Chatterjee K, Davis KB, et al. Present use of bedside right heart catheterization in patients with cardiac disease. American College of Cardiology. *J Am Coll Cardiol.* 1998;32(3):840-864.
2. Chatterjee K. The Swan-Ganz catheters: past, present, and future a viewpoint. *Circulation.* 2009;119:147-152.

CHAPTER 11

Right and Left Heart Hemodynamics

"Accuracy of statement is one of the first elements of truth; inaccuracy is a near kin to falsehood."

—Tryon Edwards

Cardiac Hemodynamics

Hemodynamic measurement is an integral part of the complete left- and right heart catheterization procedures.[1] These data help cardiologists to establish the diagnosis in many complex cases. The correct measurements and interpretation of the obtained hemodynamic data (Table 11.1) are crucial.

The normal RA waveform consists of 3 positive and 3 negative waves (Figure 11.1A). Positive waves are termed: "a", "c", and "v". The negative waves are termed: "x", "x'", and "y". The "a" wave represents atrial contraction. It can be observed around 80 ms after the peak of the "P" wave on ECG, and its amplitude depends on the strength of RA contraction and RV compliance. In general, the "a" wave is slightly higher than the following "c" wave, which normally represents the upper motion of the floor of the tricuspid valve during isovolumic RV contraction with subsequent increase of RA pressure. The "c" wave contributes to the formation of "x" and "x'" negative waves and corresponds to the "R" wave on the ECG. The "v" wave peaks normally during the last third of the "T" wave on ECG and corresponds to passive RA filling during ventricular contraction. The initial "x" wave, ending prior to the "c" wave, corresponds to RA relaxation and its early filling; on the other hand, the "x'" wave, which follows the "c" wave, corresponds to RA downward

TABLE 11.1   General rules in reading pressure tracings.

1. Identify the cardiac rhythm.
2. Determine the pressure scale.
3. Note recording speed.
4. Obtain a simultaneous ECG tracing to time the pressure tracings.
5. Interpret the waveforms in conjunction with the clinical presentation.
6. Identify common pressure artifacts such as "underdamping" or "overdamping".
7. Correctly place the transducer at zero position.

movement during early RV systolic motion. The negative "y" wave follows the positive "v" wave and corresponds to RA passive emptying into the RV during ventricular diastole. The mean RA pressure corresponds to the midpoint between the peaks of "a" and "v" and nadirs of "x'" and "y" waves. This value provides information on the right ventricular preload.

The PAW pressure tracing (Figure 11.1B) in general represents the events occurring in the LA, and reflects the same changes in LA pressure as the ones observed on RA pressure tracings described above. Transmission of the LA pressure through the pulmonary venous system causes slight (around 220 ms) delay of the PAW pressure waves in relation to directly obtained LA pressure waves and in relation to the ECG waves. So the "a" wave frequently corresponds to the "R" wave on ECG, the "c" wave to the beginning of the "T" wave, and the "v" wave, which is greater than "a", projects on a late "T-P" interval. This is usually not clinically significant, but becomes more important in simultaneous pressure measurements for mitral valve gradients. The normal RV and LV pressure tracings (Figures 11.1C and E) represent a positive, monophasic systolic wave with an occasional early systolic notch, a negative, sharp, early diastolic filling wave followed by a positive wave of passive ventricular filling, and subsequently active atrial "kick".

Interpretation of Right and Left Heart Pressure Tracings

The end-diastolic pressure is taken in the trough after the atrial "kick." Another notch can be seen on the early diastolic filling wave of the LV and RV called incisura, which represents closing of aortic and pulmonary valves. In normal conditions, the RV end-diastolic

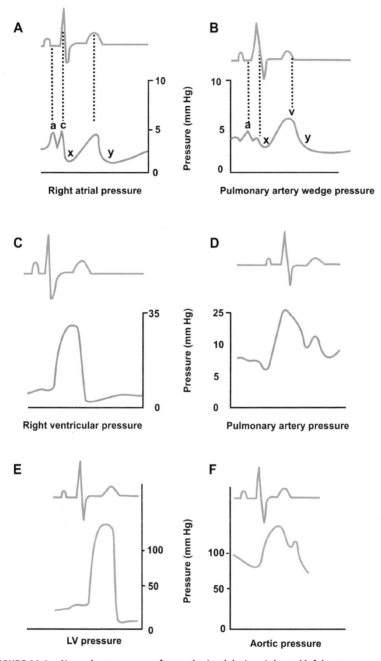

FIGURE 11.1   Normal pressure waveforms obtained during right and left heart catheterization are shown. **Panel A**: Normal RA waveform consists of 3 positive and 3 negative waves. **Panel B**: The PAW pressure tracing. **Panel C**: Normal RV pressure tracing. **Panel D**: Normal PA pressure tracing. **Panel E**: Normal LV pressure tracing. **Panel F**: Normal aortic pressure tracing.

pressure is lower than the corresponding LV end-diastolic pressure, since the RV is a more compliant chamber. The normal PA and aortic pressure tracings (Figures 11.1D and F) reflect transmitted systolic RV and LV pressures plus diastolic pressure waves, the amplitude of which depend on pulmonary and systemic vascular resistance. Under normal conditions, the PA and aortic diastolic pressures are higher than the corresponding RV and LV end-diastolic pressures, so that PA and aortic pressure tracings are characterized by transition to a smaller pulse pressure with equivalent corresponding systolic pressures.

Cardiac Output Measurement

Two of the most commonly used methods of determining cardiac output, the thermodilution method and the Fick oxygen method, are based on the principle described by Adolphus Fick in 1870, which states that the rate of delivery to or withdrawal of a substance from the circulation is equal to the product of blood flow and the difference in concentration across the point of delivery or withdrawal. Cardiac output is usually expressed in liters/minute.[2] The cardiac index (CI) equals CO divided by the patient's body surface area (BSA). Normal range of CI is 2.6–4.2 L/min/m². A CI less than 1.0 L/min/m² is generally incompatible with life.

THERMODILUTION METHOD

The pulmonary artery catheter is used to calculate CO with the thermodilution method. It contains a separate lumen for injecting saline, which terminates proximally (usually positioned in the RA) to the distal end of the catheter (Figure 11.2). The distal end of the catheter is placed in the pulmonary artery and contains the temperature sensor. Applying the Fick principle, the operator uses a fixed volume (10 mL) of cold normal saline as a substance injected smoothly but rapidly over 2–3 seconds and measures the concentration (temperature difference between saline and blood) of this substance downstream, determining CO from the concentration–time curve.

Slight variations in the injected volume will significantly alter results. Each injection should be well coordinated with the equipment. The entire process, from the point of aspiration into the injection syringe of cold normal saline to the point of its injection, should not take more than 10 seconds, since the solution warms

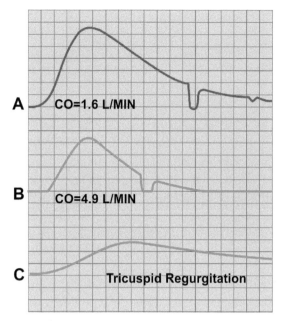

FIGURE 11.2   Cardiac output is measured by the thermodilution technique (see text for details).

by 1°C for every 28 seconds at room temperature, and the rate of warming increases if the injectate is held in a gloved hand. An operator averages the 3 best readings (variation should be less than 10%) and discounts obvious outliers. It is expected that the first CO measurement in a series will be higher than the subsequent measurements, since with the first injection, some of the indicator is lost as the catheter itself is cooled. The result is a smaller thermodilution curve, which translates into a higher CO number that generally should be discarded. Arrhythmias during injection will affect the thermodilution curve such that it is not representative of true CO, so these curves should also be discarded. The thermodilution method ideally should not be used in patients with more than mild tricuspid and/or pulmonary regurgitation and presence of intracardiac shunting.[3] It should be avoided in patients with very low cardiac output states due to a high possibility of erroneous measurements. In conditions such as significant tricuspid and/or pulmonary regurgitation, a portion of the injected cold solution volume "washes" back and forth between the RA and RV, yielding a thermodilution curve that is easily recognized by its prolonged decay time, and since the area under the thermodilution curve is inversely related to CO, the latter will be underestimated.[3] It is important to remember that the thermodilution method measures pulmonary blood flow, which is usually nearly identical in a normal state to systemic blood flow; therefore, this method is not appropriate for patients in whom left-to-right shunts exist.

FICK OXYGEN METHOD FOR CARDIAC OUTPUT MEASUREMENT

Utilizing the Fick principle and oxygen as the withdrawal substance, the following can be stated: Systemic CO equals to total O_2 consumption divided by the arteriovenous O_2 content difference (e.g., systemic arterial O_2 content minus mixed venous O_2 content). Total O_2 consumption can be directly measured or can be estimated by a formula or nomogram (see Chapter 19). Direct measurement can be achieved by either of 2 methods: One utilizes a machine designed for this purpose; the other uses a Douglas bag. Neither of these methods are free from errors, but they are still better than data derived from a formula or from a standard nomogram due to wide interpatient variability.

When using the Fick method to calculate CO, attention should be made on clinical factors that could potentially affect the measurement, such as high or low metabolic states. Ideally, one would not use the Fick method for very high cardiac output states due to its decreased reliability in such cases. Similarly, in certain conditions, such as septic shock and adult respiratory distress syndrome, the arteriovenous oxygen difference does not correlate well with CO. In addition, since the Fick method measures pulmonary flow, using it becomes a problem in patients with significant intracardiac shunting, since the pulmonary blood flow and systemic blood flow are no longer equal. On the other hand, in patients with significant mitral and/or aortic regurgitation, the total cardiac output of the LV includes both systemic flow and regurgitant blood flow, so in these situations, the pulmonary blood flow remains an accurate measure of systemic blood flow, but does not measure the volume of LV regurgitation.

Systemic arterial O_2 content equals O_2 carrying capacity multiplied by systemic arterial O_2 saturation. Mixed venous O_2 content equals O_2 carrying capacity multiplied by mixed venous O_2 saturation calculated using the Flamm formula ($3 \times$ SVC O_2sat + IVC O_2 sat)/4. The O_2 carrying capacity is the maximal amount of O_2 that can be bound by hemoglobin (Hgb). The Hgb O_2 binding constant is 1.36 mL O_2/g hemoglobin. If Hgb carrying capacity is expressed in units of mL O_2/liter blood, and Hgb concentration in the standard units of grams per deciliter, then a factor of 10 is required to adjust the units: Hgb O_2 carrying capacity = Hgb concentration $\times$ 1.36 $\times$ 10. In cases where O_2 is administered to the patient, the amount of dissolved O_2 may become significant, and it needs to be included in the calculation of O_2 content. In the absence of a shunt, samples of blood of 2–3 mL for measurement of O_2 saturation are drawn into 5-mL heparinized syringes. Usually, 3 samples are drawn from each chamber: SVC, IVC, pulmonary artery, and arterial line; the last is used also to approximate pulmonary venous O_2 saturation. Care must be taken to avoid dilution of the blood sample with too much heparinized saline solution or contamination of the blood samples with air bubbles or with blood of earlier samplings from the other chamber. It is imperative to discard the first 2 mL of blood when starting to aspirate the blood from the new chamber, and when finished with all the samples from this chamber, to flush the catheter.

Pulmonary and Systemic Vascular Resistance

Vascular resistance equals the ratio of the pressure gradient across the vascular bed to flow through the same vascular bed [PVR = (mean PAP – mean LAP)/cardiac output]. Since in most cases mean LA pressure is equal to mean PAWP, the above formula can be written in the following way: PVR = (mean PAP – mean PAWP)/cardiac output. On the other hand, SVR = (mean systemic arterial pressure – mean RAP)/cardiac output; when pressure is expressed in mm Hg and CO in L/minute, vascular resistance is expressed in Wood units. To convert into the absolute resistance units, Wood units need to be multiplied by 80. (For normal values see Chapter 19).

References

1. Wilkinson JL. Hemodynamic calculations in the catheter laboratory. *Heart.* 2001;85(113-120).
2. Hofer CK, Ganter MT, Zollinger A. What technique should I use to measure cardiac output? *Curr Opin Crit Care.* 2007;13(3):208-217.
3. Nishikawa T, Dohi S. Errors in the measurement of cardiac output by thermodilution. *Can J Anaesth.* 1993;40(2):142-153.

CHAPTER 12

Shunt Detection and Calculation

"The truth is rarely pure and never simple."

—Oscar Wilde

Oximetry for Shunt Calculations

Oximetry is the most convenient and commonly used method for detecting and calculating left-to-right shunts in the cardiac catheterization laboratory. To document the presence of the shunt and calculate its size, venous and arterial access should be obtained. Oxygen saturation is measured in SVC, IVC, RA, RV, and PA and compared with normal oxygen saturation values (see Chapter 19).[1] If femoral vein access is used for right heart catheterization, the small-diameter, 4-Fr short entry sheath is placed in the common femoral artery. The peripheral arterial line can be utilized for systemic arterial oxygen saturation measurement when jugular or subclavian veins are used as access sites for right heart catheterization. A "step-up" of mean O_2 blood saturation from SVC to PA > 7% suggests presence of an intracardiac shunt. If a steady and consistent rise > 5% in mean oxygen saturation is noted at any point while moving the PA catheter from one cardiac chamber to another, the presence of a shunt is highly suspected.

In general, when consequently performing blood oximetry from the caval veins towards the pulmonary artery, the chamber where such a "step-up" is first noted is usually the one where the shunt exists. On some occasions, a further rise in O_2 saturation occurs in the chamber distal to the initial site of a shunt as more complete mixing occurs. When a shunt is absent, pulmonary blood flow equals systemic blood flow. On the other hand, when a left-to-right shunt is present, pulmonary flow (Qp) is higher, and the ratio between Qp and systemic blood flow (Qs) can be used to character-ize the severity of the shunt. A shunt is considered small if the Qp/Qs ratio is < 1.5; it is moderate if it ranges between 1.5–2.0; and any ratio above 2.0 is considered a large shunt.

The simplicity of calculating Qp/Qs ratio is the fact that it is not necessary to calculate each of the flows separately by the Fick formula, since most of the variables and constants in this formula cancel each other out by taking the ratio. Thus, the final ratio is calculated as:

$$Qp/Qs = \frac{O_2 sat \text{ (systemic arterial)} - O_2 sat \text{ (systemic mixed venous)}}{O_2 sat \text{ (pulmonary venous)} - O_2 sat \text{ (pulmonary arterial)}}$$

To calculate systemic mixed venous O_2sat, the Flamm formula is often used:

$$O_2 sat \text{ (systemic mixed venous)} = 3 \times O_2 sat \text{ (SVC)} + O_2 sat \text{ (IVC)} / 4$$

Some physicians recommend using SVC O_2sat instead of mixed venous O_2 saturation in the presence of a suspected shunt, since the Flamm formula does not adequately compensate for the large variation in IVC O_2 saturations that may be present independent of the degree of shunting. If clinical suspicion for right-to-left shunt exists, O_2 saturation should be checked at the "wedge" position, LV, and descending aorta. The last 2 measurements can be obtained by using a 4-Fr pigtail or multipurpose catheter when cannulating the LV and the descending thoracic aorta. The presence of desaturated blood in the LV and/or descending aorta compared to the "wedge" blood sample saturation suggests a right-to-left shunt.

Blood samples for oximetry should be withdrawn into the syringe slowly, since rapid withdrawal can increase oxygen satura-tion in the sample. All samples should be taken at room air or with a gas mixture less than 30% oxygen content, since (as mentioned earlier) this may affect the saturation data and cause the shunt size to be calculated erroneously. If a bidirectional shunt is suspected, the approximate left-to-right and right-to-left shunts can be calcu-lated respectively by subtracting from Qp the hypothetical flow that would exist if no shunt were present, and from Qs the hypothetical flow that would exist if no shunt were present. This hypothetical flow can be calculated by:

$$O_2 \text{ consumption}/PV\ O_2 \text{ content} - \text{mixed venous } O_2 \text{ content}$$

Reference

1. Hillis LD, Firth BG, Winniford MD. Variability of right-sided cardiac oxygen saturations in adults with and without left-to-right intracardiac shunting. *Am J Cardiol.* 1986;58(129-132).

CHAPTER 13

Endomyocardial Biopsy

"When in doubt, abstain."

—Zoroaster

Indications and Contraindications of the Procedure

The percutaneous intravascular endomyocardial cardiac biopsy procedure using flexible bioptome was introduced by Sakakibara and Konno in 1962[1] and subsequently improved by Caves and Stinson.[2] Indications and contraindications[3-6] for the procedure are outlined in Tables 13.1 and 13.2, respectively.

The procedure is performed under mild sedation, with ECG, blood pressure, and pulse oximetry monitoring. Transthoracic 2D or 3D guidance[7] for the intracardiac bioptome tip position can be used in addition to or instead of fluoroscopic guidance, especially in pregnant patients or patients where a specific site needs to be biopsied. To access RV endomyocardium, the RIJ and the femoral vein approaches are commonly used and will be described. The femoral artery approach for accessing the LV endomyocardium will also be described. Right heart catheterization with recording of pressure tracings before and after RV endomyocardial biopsy is highly recommended. When LV endomyocardial biopsy is performed, a simultaneous right heart catheterization is advised.

TABLE 13.1   Indications for endomyocardial biopsy.

Right Ventricular Biopsy
Major Indications:
- Monitoring of cardiac allograft rejection
- Diagnosis and staging of anthracycline toxicity
- Diagnosis of certain types of myocarditis
Minor Indications:
- Diagnosis of certain types of infiltrative and inflammatory cardiomyopathies
- Diagnosis of restrictive versus constrictive heart disease
- Diagnosis of the cause of unexplained, life-threatening ventricular arrhythmias

Left Ventricular Biopsy
- Failed or nondiagnostic RV biopsy
- Diseases with selective LV involvement

TABLE 13.2   Contraindications to endomyocardial biopsy.

Absolute Contraindications
- LV thrombus when LV biopsy planned
- Aortic valve mechanical prosthesis when LV biopsy planned

Relative Contraindications
- Coagulopathy (INR > 1.5 and/or platelet count < 100,000/mL)
- RA or RV thrombus
- Recent myocardial infarction with myocardial thinning planned for biopsy
- Significant right-to-left shunt (risk of paradoxical emboli)
- Profound hemodynamic compromise
- Tachycardia
- Any prior surgery or procedure affecting passage to RV, artificial conduits
- Mechanical tricuspid valve prosthesis

Jugular Vein Approach

After jugular venous access is obtained, the operator inspects the preshaped bioptome to ensure proper function and wipes it with heparinized normal saline solution at the beginning of the procedure and then after each insertion attempt. The preshaped bioptome is handled with the thumbs and index fingers of both hands (Figure 13.1). The tip is held around 4–6 cm from the distal end with the left thumb and index finger, and the right thumb and index finger hold the bioptome 10–12 cm from the proximal end. This allows control of the forward motion and torque of the bioptome with the fingers of both hands.

The operator asks his/her assistant to hold the venous sheath while the tip of the bioptome, with closed jaws, is advanced and

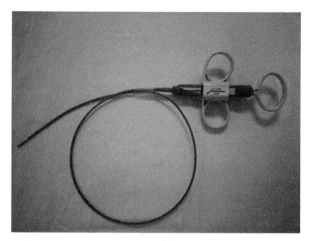

FIGURE 13.1   The endomyocardial bioptome (Argon Medical Devices, Athens, TX) is shown.

passed through it. The bioptome is advanced with the tip pointing to the patient's right (to the lateral wall of the RA) under fluoroscopic guidance, and when the tip reaches the high RA lateral
wall, the bioptome is gently torqued counterclockwise 180 degrees
using the fingers of both hands simultaneously (Figure 13.2A), then
slowly advanced through the tricuspid valve into the RV cavity
(Figure 13.2B).

If the operator feels resistance while crossing the tricuspid valve,
the bioptome should be withdrawn and another attempt made with
some change in direction. Once the bioptome tip is in the RV apex,
the operator withdraws the bioptome for 1 cm, torques it gently
counterclockwise with the fingers of both hands so that the handle
starts pointing to the posterior direction, perpendicular to the floor,
and directs the tip posteriorly towards the interventricular septum.
The plane of the septum is simulated by a 45-degree angle from
the tip of the patient's nose to the patient's right shoulder. Slight
advancement with the bioptome jaws closed is followed by a premature ventricular contraction, indicating contact with the ventricular rather than atrial endocardium. The operator obtains images
of the bioptome at PA projection, where the bioptome should be
visualized crossing the spine, its tip lying below the upper margin of
the left hemidiaphragm, and at RAO 30-degree projection followed
by LAO 60-degree projection to confirm correct position of the tip
against the midportion of the interventricular septum. These views
will help to discover unintentional positioning of the bioptome in
the coronary sinus and infradiaphragmatic vein.

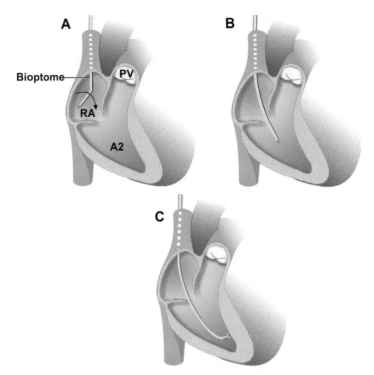

FIGURE 13.2   The jugular vein approach for endomyocardial biopsy includes the following steps: **Panel A**: The bioptome is advanced with the tip pointing to the lateral wall of the RA under fluoroscopic guidance and torqued 180 degrees. **Panel B**: The bioptome is slowly advanced through the tricuspid valve into the RV cavity. **Panel C**: Once inside the RV cavity, the bioptome jaws are opened, bioptome is advanced to engage the interventricular septum, and a biopsy is obtained.

In patients with severe RV dilatation, rotation of the heart may occur in the chest, with a portion of the RV free wall wrapping around posteriorly, and this may lead to RV free wall biopsy despite a fluoroscopically correct position of the bioptome tip. The 2D or 3D echocardiographic images can be used for final confirmation of correct location of the tip of the bioptome against the interventricular septum. The bioptome is retracted about 1 cm, and the right hand of the operator moves to the biopsy handle, while the left hand remains on the bioptome body slightly above the hub of the venous sheath. The jaws of the bioptome are opened, and the bioptome is advanced to engage the interventricular septum (Figure 13.2C). As the septal wall is engaged, the operator gently closes the bioptome jaws and withdraws the bioptome with jaws closed under fluoroscopic guidance all the way out of the sheath, with the left hand of the operator holding the sheath in place. A minor tug is felt initially when withdrawing the bioptome. In cases where excessive resistance and multiple premature ventricular contractions are observed, bioptome withdrawal should be avoided; instead, the bioptome jaws should be opened and the bioptome withdrawn and repositioned.

In general, 4 to 6 tissue samples are obtained, one of which is used for frozen section. Tissue from the open jaws of the bioptome is removed by gently rinsing with saline and quickly preserved in 10% formalin solution to reduce the amount of contraction artifact. Free-floating biopsy samples in formalin solution suggests the presence of a significant amount of fat tissue, which could be one of the signs of RV dysplasia, or indicate RV perforation with epicardial fat sampling. After the procedure is completed, fluoroscopy of the chest is performed to rule out pneumothorax. The patient should be kept in the observation unit for one hour after an uncomplicated procedure before discharge.

Femoral Vein Approach

For the femoral vein approach, a 7- to 8-Fr, 85-cm disposable-sheath system with dilator ("dog-leg" sheath with a 135-degree angle bend) is advanced over the 0.038-inch guidewire through the short entry sheath into the RA (Figure 13.3A). The dilator and the guidewire are subsequently withdrawn, which usually causes the preformed distal segment of the "dog-leg" sheath to drop into the RV. If this does not occur, the tricuspid valve is crossed with the help of the wire. If the distal end of the sheath is not ending inside the RV, then the balloon-tipped catheter can be used to navigate the biopsy sheath into the RV. After passing the distal end of the "dog-leg" sheath, the balloon-tipped catheter will be inflated and directed into the RV. The catheter is advanced across the tricuspid valve into the RV, where pressure is recorded, the balloon deflated, and the "dog-leg" sheath moved over the balloon-tipped catheter into the RV (Figure 13.3B). After positioning the sheath in the RV, the catheter is removed and the sheath is flushed with heparinized normal saline. The side port of the sheath is connected to a slow, continuous intravenous infusion to prevent clot formation inside the sheath. The sheath is repeatedly flushed after each insertion attempt of the bioptome to prevent clot formation.

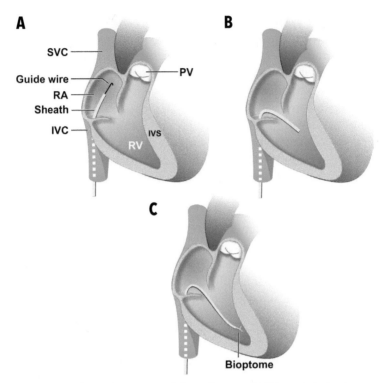

FIGURE 13.3 The femoral vein approach for endomyocardial biopsy includes the following steps: **Panel A**: A "dog-leg" sheath with a 135-degree angle bend is advanced over the 0.038-inch guidewire through the short entry sheath into the RA. **Panel B**: The dilator and the guidewire are withdrawn, causing the preformed distal segment of the "dog-leg" sheath to drop into the RV. **Panel C**: The bioptome is advanced through the "dog-leg" sheath under fluoroscopic guidance; after confirmation via imaging that the tip is against the interventricular septum, a biopsy is taken and the bioptome removed.

The distal tip of the sheath should be free-floating, directed towards the interventricular septum or posteriorly and away from the right ventricular free wall. This can be verified with 1–2 mL iodine contrast test injection under fluoroscopic guidance. The long (100 cm), unshaped, flexible bioptome is handled with the thumbs and index fingers of both hands as described for the jugular vein approach. The bioptome is gently but rapidly advanced through the "dog-leg" sheath under fluoroscopic guidance. Immediately after the tip of the bioptome passes the distal end of the sheath, the operator opens the bioptome jaws to reduce the risk of ventricular wall perforation. The operator images the bioptome at PA and LAO 60-degree projections to confirm the correct position of the tip against the interventricular septum. If the biopsy sheath is directed toward the ventricular septum, it has a posterior orientation in deep LAO view. The 2D or 3D echocardiographic images can be used for final confirmation of the correct location of the tip of the bioptome against the interventricular septum.

As the septal wall is engaged, the operator gently closes the bioptome jaws and removes the bioptome under fluoroscopic guidance out of the sheath (Figure 13.3C). The rest of the procedure is routine and is described with the jugular vein approach.

Femoral Artery Approach

There are two slightly different methods of positioning the long (90 cm), 7- to 8-Fr, curved or straight (used to biopsy left ventricular apex) sheath through the common femoral artery into the LV cavity (Figure 13.4).

FIRST OPTION

Once arterial access is obtained, the operator advances the angled pigtail catheter until it is placed in the LV cavity, where it is stabilized in the mid-ventricular position coaxial with the longitudinal axis of the LV. The tip of the exchange wire is left in the left ventricular cavity, while the pigtail catheter is removed; the preformed LV long biopsy sheath is then advanced over the wire into the LV under fluoroscopic guidance. The wire is removed, and the side port of the sheath is connected to the pressure monitoring system. After the position of the sheath in the LV is documented, the distal tip of the sheath should be free-floating, not buried into the ventricular wall, and pointed towards the interventricular septum; this can be assured with a 3- to 4-mL iodine contrast injection under fluoroscopic guidance at 45-degree LAO projection. The sheath is flushed with heparinized normal saline, LV systolic and end-diastolic pressures measured and recorded on 200 mm Hg and 50 mm Hg scales) accordingly. Flushing of the sheath is repeated after each insertion attempt of the bioptome to prevent clot formation inside the long sheath.

SECOND OPTION

Once arterial access is obtained, the operator advances the long, curved sheath over the 0.038-inch, J-tip exchange guidewire to the

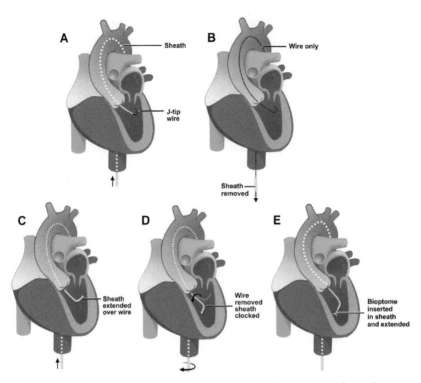

FIGURE 13.4 Diagram shows the steps of endomyocardial biopsy using a femoral artery approach. **Panel A**: The angled pigtail catheter is placed over the exchange guidewire into the LV cavity. **Panel B**: The exchange guidewire remains in the LV cavity while the pigtail catheter is removed. **Panel C**: The preformed LV long biopsy sheath is then advanced over the wire into the LV and the wire is removed subsequently. **Panel D**: The sheath is turned and pointed towards the interventricular septum. **Panel E**: After the bioptome has been advanced out of the sheath the jaws of the bioptome are opened in order to engage the interventricular septum upon further advancement.

aorta under fluoroscopic guidance, keeping the tip of the wire protruding beyond the tip of the sheath. Once the tip of the guidewire advances around the aortic arch, it gets fixed above the coronary sinus. With the tip of the sheath remaining below the aortic arch in the descending aorta, a regular, long, 6-Fr pigtail or multipurpose catheter slides over the wire until the tip of the wire is covered by the tip of the catheter. The aortic valve is crossed, and when the catheter tip is in the LV cavity, it is stabilized in the mid-ventricular position coaxial with the longitudinal axis of the LV. The catheter tip should not contact the ventricular wall or the mitral valve–chordal apparatus. When this is achieved, a preformed LV long biopsy sheath is advanced over the catheter into the LV under fluoroscopic guidance. Subsequently, the wire and the catheter are removed, and the side port of the sheath is connected to the manifold. The rest of the procedure is routine and is described above.

Before proceeding further, the operator injects 40 U/kg of heparin intravenously to keep the ACT >200 seconds, inspects the 6-Fr Stanford LV long (100 cm) bioptome (Scholten Surgical Instruments, Inc., Lodi, CA) to ensure it is functioning properly, and wipes it with heparinized normal saline solution at the beginning of the procedure and then after each insertion attempt. The handling of the bioptome is described above. The bioptome is gently advanced through the preshaped sheath under fluoroscopic guidance. Immediately after the tip of the bioptome passes the distal end of the sheath, the operator opens the bioptome jaws to reduce the risk of ventricular wall perforation. The operator images the bioptome at LAO 45-degree projection to confirm the correct position of the tip against the interventricular septum. As the LV wall is engaged, the operator gently closes the bioptome jaws and withdraws the bioptome out of the sheath. After the procedure is completed, the arterial sheath is cannulated with a long, J-tip exchange wire and exchanged over the wire to the same French short arterial sheath, and femoral angiography is performed. If a closure device can be placed, the arterial access site is closed, and the patient is kept in the observation unit for 2 hours after an uncomplicated procedure before discharge. If the closure device cannot be placed, the sheath is removed and hemostasis achieved with manual pressure. In this case, the patient's discharge time from the observation unit depends on the diameter of the arterial sheath used.

WHAT IF AN OPERATOR ENCOUNTERS ONE OF THE FOLLOWING PROBLEMS?

Perforation of Heart Chambers

RA, RV, or LV perforations (see also Chapter 10) rarely occur during endomyocardial biopsy in a cardiac catheterization laboratory where fluoroscopic and echocardiographic guidance are used. In patients with a recent heart transplant, the atrial suture line increases the risk of perforation. The risk of cardiac tamponade is significantly less in patients post cardiac transplantation or with a history of prior cardiac surgery due to presence of pericardial adhesions to the right ventricular free wall.

Arrhythmia

As the bioptome enters the cardiac chamber, the primary complications are various arrhythmias (see also Chapter 10). These arrhythmias are caused, in most cases, by the contact of the tip of the bioptome with the endocardium, and can be easily terminated by withdrawal of the bioptome. In some cases, touching the ventricular endocardial surface with the tip of the bioptome can terminate sustained ventricular tachycardia not responding to withdrawal of the bioptome.

In the presence of a baseline complete RBBB, the development of a LBBB during LV biopsy can occur. In case of delayed onset of an escape rhythm, touching the RV endocardium with the tip of the bioptome can cause mechanically induced ventricular depolarizations supporting circulation until a steady, temporarily paced rhythm is established. It should also be remembered that bradyarrhythmic episodes in heart transplant patients may respond to beta-1 mimetic agents but not to atropine.

Damage to Adjacent Structures

Endomyocardial biopsy can lead to significant tricuspid or mitral regurgitation secondary to damage of the chordal or papillary muscle apparatus. Postbiopsy echocardiographic examination can help to identify this complication in early stages. Occasionally, deep sampling may lead to resection of a branch of a major epicardial coronary artery with creation of a coronary–ventricular fistula, which in most cases is not clinically significant. Other complications include perforation of the major blood vessels such as the vena cava with inadvertent entrance into the pleural or mediastinal space, which in most cases will require surgery.

Embolism

Thromboembolism or air embolism can occur but are rare. Systemic heparinization and aspirin decrease the risk of cerebrovascular embolism.

References

1. Sakakibara S, Konno S. Endomyocardial biopsy. *Jpn Heart J.* 1962;3:537-543.

2. Caves PK, Stinson EB, Graham AF, Billingham ME, Grehl TM, Shumway NE. Percutaneous transvenous endomyocardial biopsy. *JAMA.* 1973;225(3):288-291.

3. Thiene G, Bruneval P, Veinot J, Leone O. Diagnostic use of the endomyocardial biopsy: a consensus statement. *Virchows Arch.* 2013;463(1):1-5.

4. Leone O, Veinot JP, Angelini A, et al. 2011 consensus statement on endomyocardial biopsy from the Association for European Cardiovascular Pathology and the Society for Cardiovascular Pathology. *Cardiovasc Pathol.* 2012;21(4):245-274.

5. From AM, Maleszewski JJ, Rihal CS. Current status of endomyocardial biopsy. *Mayo Clin Proc.* 2011;86(11):1095-1102.

6. Cooper LT, Baughman KL, Feldman AM, et al. The role of endomyocardial biopsy in the management of cardiovascular disease: a scientific statement from the American Heart Association, the American College of Cardiology, and the European Society of Cardiology. Endorsed by the Heart Failure Society of America and the Heart Failure Association of the European Society of Cardiology. *Circulation.* 2007;116:2216-2233.

7. Amitai ME, Schnittger I, Popp RL, Chow J, Brown P, Liang DH. Comparison of three-dimensional echocardiography to two-dimensional echocardiography and fluoroscopy for monitoring of endomyocardial biopsy. *Am J Cardiol.* 2007;99:864-866.

CHAPTER 14

Pericardiocentesis

"Speed is good when wisdom leads the way."

—Edward Roscoe Murrow

Indications and Contraindications of the Procedure

The first needle pericardiocentesis was performed in 1840 by Franz Schuh, a physician from Vienna.[1] The indications and contraindications for the procedure are outlined in Tables 14.1 and 14.2, accordingly.

No absolute contraindications exist for the emergent procedure if it is performed with the purpose of treating cardiac tamponade. If pericardiocentesis is not emergent, performing right heart catheterization with recording of pressure tracings before and after pericardiocentesis is highly recommended. The ideal site of the needle entry characteristics are the maximal diameter of the fluid layer, the shortest distance to the fluid layer, and no vital structures in the needle path from the site of entry to the pericardial space.[2]

Pericardiocentesis can be done "blindly," but it is preferable to use ECG, fluoroscopy, or ideally, echocardiography for guidance.[3] Real-time cardiac ultrasound imaging allows the operator to choose the access site, avoid liver- and lung-tissue injury, measure the distance from the point of skin entrance of the needle to the pericardium, track the trajectory of the needle tip and assure its correct location by injecting agitated normal saline into the pericardial space for opacification. Echocardiography also allows the operator to assess the cardiac response to drainage and measure the volume of the residual pericardial content after the procedure. Although in case of an emergency the procedure can be performed

TABLE 14.1   Indications for pericardiocentesis.

- Treatment of cardiac tamponade
- Evaluation and treatment of pericardial effusion

TABLE 14.2   Contraindications to pericardiocentesis.

Relative Contraindications:
- Coagulopathy (INR > 1.8, PTT > 2× normal and/or platelet count < 50,000/mL)
- Traumatic hemopericardium
- Subacute cardiac free wall rupture
- Small or posteriorly located effusions
- Purulent, grossly infected pericardial effusion
- Type A aortic dissection

at the patient's bedside; it is best done in the cardiac catheterization laboratory, where cardiac hemodynamics can be recorded. The procedure should be performed after appropriate consent is obtained from the patient, followed by mild sedation, with continuous ECG, blood pressure, and pulse oximetry monitoring.

Subxiphoid Approach

This is the most commonly used approach. The operator positions the patient at a 30- to 45-degree angle to assist with inferior pooling of fluid. The patient is asked to take shallow breaths in order to avoid significant movement of the diaphragm. The patient's subxiphoid area is surgically draped under sterile conditions. The needle access site is 1–1.5 cm below the left costoxiphoid junction (Figure 14.1).

The skin and superficial tissue over the access site is anesthetized with a 25-gauge needle containing 5 mL of 1% warm lidocaine solution. To cover the anticipated access needle path, a 22-gauge needle and an additional 10 mL of the anesthetic are needed. The access needle utilized for pericardiocentesis is marked by a sterile marker at the approximate distance between the skin and pericardial effusion as measured by echocardiography. After the tissue at the access site is well anesthetized, an 18-gauge access needle connected to a 10-mL syringe (with 2 mL of 1% lidocaine) through a 3-way stopcock, is inserted and advanced at 30- to 45-degree angle through the skin towards the posterior aspect of the left shoulder under constant aspiration. Some physicians utilize the Polytef-sheathed

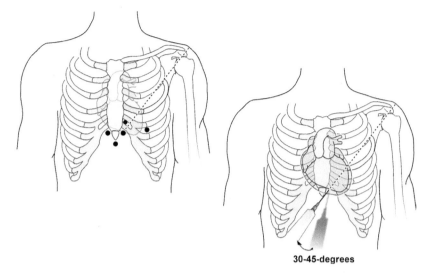

30-45-degrees

FIGURE 14.1   Diagram shows pericardiocentesis via the subxiphoid approach.

needle.[4] Upon entering the pericardial space, the Polytef sheath is advanced over the needle into the pericardial space and the needle withdrawn; the J-tip guidewire subsequently runs through the Polytef sheath and not through the needle. The operator may feel a discrete "pop" as the needle crosses the pericardium and enters the pericardial space, and back flow of pericardial fluid into the syringe is established. The needle is fixed and a second 10-mL syringe with 8 mL agitated saline mixed with 1 mL of air is attached to the 3-way stopcock, followed by injection into the pericardial space under echocardiographic visualization. If the needle tip is in the pericardial space, the injection of agitated saline will cause its opacification. In cases where the needle tip is in the RV cavity, the agitated saline will be quickly washed away by blood flow. Occasionally, due to a large pericardial effusion, injection of agitated saline might not be visible from certain echocardiographic views, so the view should be changed and the injection repeated. If fluoroscopic guidance is used, the needle position is confirmed with injection of contrast media. After making sure that position of the needle is correct, the syringe is disconnected from the needle and the 0.035-inch, J-tip guidewire is inserted and advanced through the needle into the pericardial space under fluoroscopic guidance. As the wire enters into the pericardial space, it will wrap around the heart. The needle is then removed, and a small nick of the skin is made with a scalpel at the level of guidewire entrance in order to ease the insertion of the 7- or 8-Fr dilator over the wire into the pericardial space. After the dilator is removed, the pericardiocentesis 7- or 8-Fr pigtail catheter is advanced over the guidewire into the pericardial space, and the guidewire is removed. The operator ensures that fluid return persists by aspirating it to a syringe connected to the hub of the catheter through the 3-way stopcock. Then the syringe is detached and the pressure tubing is attached to simultaneously record the pericardial pressure and the pressures from PAW, PA, RV, and RA sites. After these recordings are obtained, the pericardial pressure tubing is detached, a 60 mL syringe is reattached to the 3-way stopcock, and fluid is actively aspirated and redirected to the collecting bag, followed by gravity draining. The pericardial catheter is fixed to the skin with a couple of sutures and sterile dressing is applied. Fluoroscopy and chest x-ray are checked to exclude pneumothorax after completion of the procedure.

If an attempt to access the pericardial space with the needle is unsuccessful, the needle is withdrawn slowly, flushed, redirected, and another attempt is made. If 3 unsuccessful attempts are made, another approach should be utilized if possible. Otherwise surgical drainage is recommended. Every 24 hours for the next 48 to 72 hours, strict recording of the drainage volume is necessary. The drain should be aspirated and, if needed, flushed with sterile normal saline every 4–6 hours to ensure that the catheter is not obstructed and clotted. When and if the drainage volume becomes less than 30 mL/24 hours, the drainage catheter can be pulled. When pulling the drainage catheter, the operator should first ask the patient to take a breath and pull the catheter, during exhalation. At the end of exhalation, the patient is instructed to hold breathing, and an airtight dressing is placed across the access site. If the drainage rate remains higher, or if fluid becomes purulent, the catheter should be removed and surgical pericardial drainage pursued. Open surgical drainage offers several advantages, including complete drainage of the pericardial content, access to pericardial tissue for histopathologic and microbiologic diagnoses, the ability to drain loculated effusions and posterior effusions.

Apical Approach

The patient is placed supine with the head elevated at a 30- to 45-degree angle with a minor tilt towards left lateral decubitus position, and the left arm is positioned under the head. The needle access site and direction is dictated by real-time echocardiography. In general, the direction of the needle is towards the right shoulder tip. The rest of the technique and postprocedural management is identical to the subxiphoid approach as described.

WHAT IF AN OPERATOR ENCOUNTERS ONE OF THE FOLLOWING PROBLEMS?

Perforation of Heart Chamber

RA, RV, or LV perforation occur rarely during pericardiocentesis in a cardiac catheterization laboratory where fluoroscopic and echocardiographic guidance are actively used (see Chapter 10). The needle puncture site is usually self-sealing in the absence of coagulopathy.

Arterial Laceration

Arterial lacerations of the LAD with the apical approach, LIMA with the parasternal approach, and PDA with the subxiphoid approach are major complications, which can be easily recognized when the straw-colored pericardial fluid suddenly turns red with high O_2 saturation. The cardiothoracic surgery team should be notified to proceed with emergent surgery if the patient's hemodynamic status continues to deteriorate despite active aspiration of blood from the pericardial space and administration of intravenous fluids. Otherwise, after coronary and IMA angiography is completed and the laceration site is identified, endovascular repair can be attempted with a covered stent.

Occasionally, angiography does not reveal any source of arterial bleeding as suggested by high O_2 saturations of blood obtained from drainage. High O_2 saturation in pericardial fluid can be observed in patients with effusive constrictive pericarditis, especially if a relatively stiff wire was used to support advancement of the drainage catheter through the relatively rigid pericardial wall. This is caused by the presence of small arterial vessels in vascularized pericardial adhesions, which can get damaged during wire manipulations in the pericardial space. The reason for occasionally using a stiff wire is to better support the drainage catheter, which may start buckling at the entrance site of the rigid pericardial wall, especially if the wall was not well predilated with a dilator, causing loss of access. In such circumstance, the operator uses 1- or 2-Fr higher dilators than the drainage catheter to prevent the problem from reoccurring.

FRANK BLOOD OR BLOODY FLUID?

The operator frequently deals with this question. Several simple features can help with differentiation. First, place several mL of obtained pericardial fluid on a gauze pad and in a small bowl. Pericardial fluid creates a yellowish/pinkish halo stain around the central red stain, whereas true blood homogenously stains the gauze red. Blood from a cardiac chamber clots, while pericardial bloody fluid does not due to defibrination, which occurs after blood is in the pericardial space for a prolonged period. The presence of arterial blood can be proven by measurement of O_2 saturation and hematocrit content of the obtained fluid.

Pneumothorax

For discussion of this complication, please review the discussion of access complications in Chapter 5.

Left or Right Ventricular Systolic Dysfunction

This complication of pericardiocentesis is rare, but is well documented. It is mostly observed in patients who have large, chronic pericardial effusions, and it occurs when pericardiocentesis leads to rapid removal of large volume of pericardial fluid.[5]

The mechanism of this phenomenon is not entirely clear. The following possible hypotheses have been suggested: chronic diffuse ischemia with transient myocardial stunning; sudden increase in venous return with reverse Bernheim effect in addition to increased systemic vascular resistance secondary to hyperadrenergic state; and unmasking of underlying ventricular systolic dysfunction. In most cases, this condition is reversible. Treatment includes intravenous diuresis, vasodilator therapy, and inotropic support.

References

1. Kilpatrick ZM, Carleton BC. On pericardiocentesis. *Am J Card.* 1965;16:722-728.

2. Loukas M, Walters A, Boon JM, Welch TP, Meiring JH, Abrahams PH. Pericardiocentesis: a clinical anatomy review. *Clin Anat.* 2012;25(7):872-881.

3. Tsang TS, Freeman WK, Sinak LJ, Seward JB. Echocardiographically guided pericardiocentesis: evolution and state-of-the-art technique. *Mayo Clin Proc.* 1998;73(7):647-652.

4. Fitch MT, Nicks BA, Pariyadath M, McGinnis HD, Manthey DE. Videos in clinical medicine. Emergency pericardiocentesis. *N Engl J Med.* 2012;366(12):e17.

5. Chamoun A, Cenz R, Mager A, et al. Acute left ventricular failure after large volume pericardiocentesis. *Clin Cardiol.* 2003;26(12):588-590.

CHAPTER 15

Intra-Aortic Balloon Pump (IABP) Placement

"The expectations of life depend upon diligence; the mechanic that would perfect his work must first sharpen his tools."

—Confucius

Indications and Contraindications of the Procedure

The percutaneous method of insertion of an intra-aortic balloon pump (IABP) through the femoral artery was introduced in 1979[1] and is performed usually in a cardiac catheterization laboratory, where optimal placement can be guided by fluoroscopy.[2,3] Indications and contraindications for the procedure are outlined in Tables 15.1 and 15.2, accordingly.

Femoral Artery Approach

The right or left common femoral artery often serve as access sites of choice; on rare occasions, the left brachial access can be considered (Figure 15.1A). The balloon size is based on patient's height: Patients taller than 183 cm receive 50-mL balloons, patients less than 162 cm receive 30-mL balloons, and all other patients receive 40-mL balloons. The balloon diameter, when fully expanded, should not exceed 80%–90% of the diameter of the descending aorta.

TABLE 15.1   Indications for intra-aortic balloon pump placement.

- Cardiogenic shock
- Acute severe mitral regurgitation
- Acute severe ventricular septal defect
- Refractory ischemia
- High-risk PCI

TABLE 15.2   Contraindications to intra-aortic balloon pump placement.

- Severe coagulopathy
- Aortic dissection
- Aortic regurgitation ($\geq$ moderate)
- Significant arteriovenous shunts
- Sepsis
- No plans for definitive therapy
- Large thoracic or thoracoabdominal aneurysm
- Large abdominal aortic aneurysm (relative, can still use left brachial access in patients with focal infrarenal AAA)
- Severe bilateral low extremity peripheral vascular disease (relative, can still use left brachial access)
- Femoro-popliteal bypass grafts

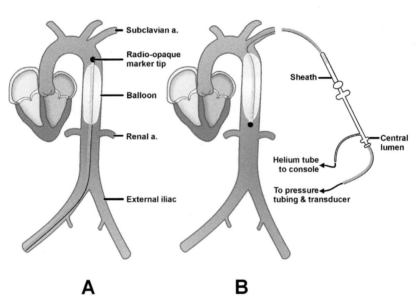

FIGURE 15.1   Optimal positioning of the IABP is shown in (Panel A) the femoral artery approach and **(Panel B)** the left brachial artery approach.

As the tip of the needle is in the lumen of the common femoral artery, the 0.030-inch or 0.032-inch, J-tip guidewire is inserted and advanced through the needle into the descending aorta. Once the 7.5-Fr sheath is appropriately positioned, the side port of the sheath is connected to the manifold to record arterial pressure. A 60-mL syringe is connected to the balloon port, and the plunger of the syringe is slowly and completely withdrawn to create a vacuum within the balloon in order to minimize its bulk at insertion. The IABP central lumen is flushed with heparin, and it is advanced over the guidewire through the arterial sheath under fluoroscopic guidance into the aorta so that the radiopaque marker tip lies about 2 cm below the origin of the left subclavian artery or at the level of the carina, with the distal end above the renal arteries (usually corresponds to L1–L2 vertebrae). There should be no resistance to passing the balloon. Resistance usually indicates aorto-iliac disease, and in this case the balloon should be withdrawn and the aorto-iliac segment reassessed by angiography. Inflation of the balloon in this position should not cause occlusion of either the renal or subclavian arteries. The guidewire is withdrawn; the central lumen is aspirated and flushed with heparinized saline, and is attached to a pressure transducer.

The operator connects the balloon inflation port of the IABP catheter to the IABP console and fills the balloon with helium gas. The balloon should unwrap fully and there should be no kinks or filling defects. Complete filling of the balloon and its position should be verified by fluoroscopy. At this point, a cine image is obtained, and the angiographic frame stored.

When all these steps are completed, counterpulsation is initiated. A heparin bolus at 40 units/kg is given intravenously and a drip started at 12 units/kg/hour to keep PTT at 1.5-times control to reduce the incidence of thromboembolism. Distal pulses are checked, the proximal end is sutured securely to the skin and sterile dressing is applied. While the balloon is in position, the patient remains on strict bed rest with no hip flexion beyond 20 degrees. To obtain maximum hemodynamic effect from counterpulsation, it is crucial to optimally adjust the timing of balloon inflation and deflation. When adjusting timing of the balloon inflation and deflation, the operator places the balloon on a 1:2 counterpulsation sequence and observes the arterial waveforms of augmented and unaugmented beats from the catheter's central lumen. Balloon inflation should immediately follow the closure of the aortic valve, coinciding with the dicrotic notch on the central aortic pressure tracing.

Balloon deflation should be set to occur immediately prior to the aortic valve opening, which usually coincides with the "R" wave on the ECG tracing. Pacing spikes should be used to trigger the balloon in patients who are 100% paced. If the balloon functions well and timing is set correctly, the augmentation wave should be greater than the systolic pressure, and postdeflation aortic end-diastolic pressure should be 10–15 mm Hg lower than the same parameter of a nonaugmented beat (Figure 15.2C). After IABP insertion, peripheral pulses on both lower extremities must be checked regularly and frequently, and daily chest x-rays and general laboratory values (CBC, serum electrolytes, PTT) should be obtained.

Left Brachial Artery Approach

As mentioned above, if needed and no contraindications exist, the IABP can be placed from the left brachial approach (Figure 15.1B).[4] If passage of the guidewire meets with resistance, the operator is advised, after placing a 4- to 5-Fr sheath, to deploy the straight pigtail catheter and perform angiography to define the left subclavian and brachial anatomy prior to the decision to place the IABP. Otherwise, the 4- to 5-Fr sheath is exchanged over the guidewire to a 7.5-Fr IABP sheath. Heparin bolus of 40 units/kg should be administered intravenously as soon as access is obtained in order to avoid arterial sheath thrombosis. The IABP is advanced over the guidewire through the hemostatic one-way valve of the arterial sheath under fluoroscopic guidance into the descending aorta so that the radiopaque marker tip lies above the renal arteries, which usually corresponds to L1–L2 vertebrae, and with the proximal end of the balloon about 2 cm below the origin of the left subclavian artery at the level of the carina. Occasionally, the guidewire tends to go toward the ascending aorta in this case an internal mammary catheter can be used to navigate the guidewire towards the descending aorta and then exchanged with the IABP. There should be no resistance to passing the balloon; resistance usually indicates aorto-subclavian disease, and the balloon should be withdrawn and the aorto-subclavian segment assessed by angiography. Inflation of the balloon should not cause occlusion of either the renal or subclavian arteries. The subsequent steps are identical to the femoral approach and have been described previously. While the balloon is in position the patient's left arm remains straight; the patient's head can be raised to 30 degrees.

Occasionally, the operator may decide to use sheathless insertion of the IABP, especially in smaller patients, in patients with peripheral arterial disease, or when the left brachial approach is utilized. However, disadvantages of sheathless insertion include the inability to reposition the IABP once placed and a greater potential to become infected from skin flora.

Cardiac catheterization can be safely performed by transiently turning the balloon off during all catheter exchanges in order to prevent the diagnostic catheter tip from perforating the balloon.

Removal of the IABP is done after successful weaning from counterpulsation. The weaning process starts by decreasing the counterpulsation rate from 1:1 to 1:2 while the patient is closely observed for several hours. If the patient remains hemodynamically stable, further decrease in rate is performed down to 1:3 for an hour, and if patient continues to remain stable, the rate is decreased to 1:4 for a short period prior to removal. The heparin drip is stopped, and when ACT becomes less than 170 seconds, the operator proceeds with pump removal. The area of the skin and underlying soft tissue around the site of the femoral sheath entry is infiltrated with 15–20 mL 1% lidocaine in order to decrease the discomfort associated with balloon removal, and consequently to reduce the chance of vagal reaction developing in association with pain. Continuous ECG and monitoring of O_2 saturation and BP is highly recommended. Good peripheral venous access, combined with a fluid bag of normal saline and 1 mg of atropine at the patient's bedside, are necessary to treat possible profound vagal reaction.

When all preparations are completed the operator turns off the pump, connects a 60-mL syringe to the central catheter lumen, and withdraws all the helium out of the balloon in order to completely deflate it. The balloon cannot be withdrawn through the sheath; rather, the balloon and sheath are removed as one unit. The operator cuts the fixing sutures first, places the right hand over the site of femoral (left brachial) access in such manner that the index finger is positioned below the site of entry of the sheath, and applies occlusive pressure on the distal segment of the femoral (left brachial) artery. Meanwhile, the middle finger is placed above the site of entry following the path of femoral (left brachial) artery. Using the other hand, the operator withdraws the balloon and sheath as one unit through the site, and allows the puncture site to bleed freely for a few seconds while keeping distal pressure with the index finger. Then the operator applies proximal occlusive pressure on the artery and releases the distal pressure for a few seconds to allow back-bleeding. The operator then reapplies distal pressure and continues applying proximal pressure on the artery for the next 15 minutes with frequent monitoring of the distal pulses during manual compression.

It is important to be meticulous in the process of removing the intra-aortic balloon pump in order to avoid distal embolization of thrombi, which may form on the balloon catheter and near the insertion site. A sterile dressing is applied to the site after hemostasis has been achieved and the patient is kept at strict bed rest (femoral access; not required for left brachial access), under close observation of the access site, and frequent (every 15 minutes for the first hour, once per hour for 2 hours and then every 4 hours) assessment of distal pulses for 8 hours.

SO WHAT IF AN OPERATOR ENCOUNTERS ONE OF THE FOLLOWING PROBLEMS?

Suboptimal Timing of IABP Inflation and Deflation

Four possible versions of suboptimal IABP timing (Figure 15.2A–E) can occur:

- **Early inflation:** Inflation of the balloon occurs before the dicrotic notch, which can potentially lead to early closure of the aortic valve, increased afterload, LV wall stress and oxygen consumption, and drop of stroke volume. On pressure tracing, blurring from unassisted systole and assisted diastole is noted. To correct the problem, the inflation time should be slightly delayed so that the dicrotic notch becomes visible and then set back until correct timing of the inflation is reached, which can be judged by the inflation coinciding with the dicrotic notch and by transition to a normal IABP pressure tracing.
- **Delayed inflation:** Inflation of the balloon occurs after the dicrotic notch, which can potentially lead to suboptimal coronary perfusion. On pressure tracing, diastolic augmentation is not adequate, with assisted diastolic pressure wave amplitude less than unassisted systolic wave. To correct the problem, the inflation time should be set slightly earlier so the dicrotic notch becomes first invisible and then moved forward until correct timing of inflation is reached. This can be judged by the presence of a normal IABP pressure tracing.
- **Early deflation:** Early deflation may lead to suboptimal coronary perfusion, increased afterload due to deflation of the balloon

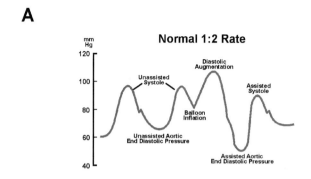

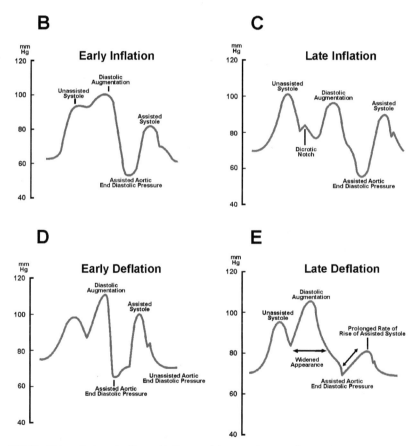

FIGURE 15.2 Timing of inflation/deflation of the IABP (see text for details). **Panel A**: Normal aortic blood pressure tracing with optimal inflation of the IABP. **Panel B**: Abnormal aortic blood pressure tracing with early inflation of the IABP. **Panel C**: Abnormal aortic blood pressure tracing with late inflation of the IABP. **Panel D**: Abnormal aortic blood pressure tracing with early deflation of the IABP. **Panel E**: Abnormal aortic blood pressure tracing with late deflation of the IABP.

before the isovolumic contraction phase of the left ventricle, and increased myocardial oxygen demand. On pressure tracing, it can be recognized as a precipitous drop of the augmented diastolic pressure to numbers less than expected and the assisted systolic pressure amplitude higher than unassisted systolic pressure. To correct the problem, the deflation time should be set later, until correct timing of deflation is reached, which can be judged by transition to a normal IABP pressure tracing.

- **Delayed deflation:** Delayed deflation leads to increased early systolic aortic pressure due to the fact that ventricular ejection may begin against an incompletely deflated balloon, which may cause increased afterload, LV wall stress, oxygen demand, and reduced stroke volume. The pressure tracing shows the assisted end-diastolic pressure amplitude equal to or greater than unassisted end-diastolic pressure, a prolonged rate of rise of the assisted systole, and widened diastolic augmentation. To correct the problem, the deflation time should be set earlier, until correct timing of deflation is reached, which can be judged by transition to a normal IABP pressure tracing.

Sepsis and Confirmed Bacteremia

The IABP should be removed and the infection treated appropriately.

Thrombocytopenia and Hemolysis

Platelet count usually does not drop below 50,000/mL and recovers quickly after pumping is stopped. If this does not occur, other causes of thrombocytopenia should be investigated. Severe hemolysis secondary to IABP is rare, and will require balloon removal.

Cerebrovascular Accident

Cerebrovascular accident is a rare complication of the IABP. An operator needs to make sure that the position of the balloon is not proximal to the subclavian artery, there is no rupture of the balloon, and there is no extensive retrograde dissection of the aortic arch.

Limb Ischemia and Distal Embolization

Pre-existing arterial disease with severe narrowing of the internal diameter of the common femoral or iliac artery may lead to mechanical obstruction of the vessel by the 7.5-Fr IABP system with limb ischemia, occurring soon after balloon insertion. When this is noted, the balloon pump should be removed and an attempt made to place it in the contralateral leg. If limb ischemia is not resolved, vascular surgery needs to be promptly contacted.

Thrombosis

Local thrombosis occurs mostly in the presence of local athero-sclerotic disease, but may also occur with local arterial dissection. When this is noted the balloon pump should be removed and an attempt made to place it in the contralateral leg. If limb ischemia has not resolved, vascular surgery needs to be promptly contacted.

Vessel Dissection

Vessel dissection can occur in the aorta or the iliac or femoral arteries, and can be caused at the time of balloon insertion or as a result of balloon inflation. Most of these dissections are downstream to the blood flow, and unless they create organ or limb ischemia, should be managed by IABP removal and observation, otherwise vascular surgery needs to be promptly contacted.

Distal Embolization

Balloon rupture occurs rarely and can vary from a very small leak to a catastrophic rupture (see Chapter 17). The usual causes are mishandling of the balloon during insertion, or balloon erosion secondary to calcified plaque. Usually, the balloon pump picks up the leak and gives a signal, but an operator should always be vigilant and check the extracorporeal tubing for presence of blood, especially if a sudden change in diastolic waveform is noted. When this is discovered, pumping should be immediately stopped and the balloon removed. Otherwise, helium embolization with catastrophic consequences to a patient can occur. The massive blood clotting inside the balloon will inevitably lead to surgical removal of the balloon. If the presence of an "entrapped clotted balloon" is recognized in less than one hour, an attempt can be made to inject t-PA into the gas-driven lumen of the IABP in an attempt to dissolve the clot and enable normal percutaneous removal of the IABP in order to avoid surgery.[5,6]

Arrhythmia

Arrhythmias can affect proper timing of inflation and deflation of the IABP. With rates greater than 120–130 bpm, the operator may consider switching IABP to the 1:2 counterpulsation mode, especially with older type balloon pumps which cannot fill and empty fast enough, to improve the efficiency of hemodynamic support.

Pre-Existing Grafts

Artificial (Dacron) aorto-femoral or ileo-femoral grafts can be used as percutaneous access site for the placement of an IABP. The graft access site needs to be appropriately prepared to be able to accommodate the 7.5-Fr sheath. When the access needle goes through the Dacron graft, the operator will not feel the sudden drop of the needle tip into the graft cavity; rather, the constant "grip" of the graft on the needle will be felt as soon as the needle tip goes through the graft.

When the access needle is in the graft cavity a pulsatile blood return should be observed. The rest of the steps are routine and are described earlier in detail. The only difference is in using an 8-Fr dilator first to go in-and-out over the guidewire through the graft, followed by sheath deployment. This maneuver prepares the graft access to be able to accommodate the 7.5-Fr IABP sheath. When removing the IABP through the Dacron graft, full compression of the graft should be avoided at all times, due to an increased risk of graft thrombosis. Sufficient pressure for prevention of the bleeding should be applied. If this complication still occurs, a vascular surgeon should be consulted without delay.

References

1. Bergman HE, Casarella WJ. Percutaneous intra-aortic balloon pumping: initial clinical experience. *Ann Thorac Surg.* 1980;29:153-155.
2. De Waha S, Desch S, Eitel I, et al. Intra-aortic balloon counterpulsation — basic principles and clinical evidence. *Vascul Pharmacol.* 2014;60(2):52-56.
3. Trost JC, Hillis LD. Intra-aortic balloon counterpulsation. *Am J Cardiol.* 2006;97(9):1391-1398.
4. Aznaouridis K, Kacharava AG, Consolini M, Zafari AM, Mavromatis K. Transbrachial intra-aortic balloon pumping for high-risk percutaneous coronary intervention. *Am J Med Sci.* 2011;341(2):153-156.
5. Fitzmaurice GJ, Collins A, Parissis H. Management of intra-aortic balloon pump entrapment. *Tex Heart Inst J.* 2012;39(5):621-626.
6. Fukushima Y, Yoshioka M, Hirayama N, Kashiwagi T, Onitsuka T, Koga Y. Management of intra-aortic balloon entrapment. *Ann Thorac Surg.* 1995;60(4):1109-1111.

Temporary Transvenous Pacemaker Placement

"What we hope ever to do with ease we must learn first to do with diligence."

—Samuel Johnson

Indications and Contraindications of the Procedure

Placement of a temporary transvenous pacemaker[1] can be achieved by employing any of the described central venous approaches (Figure 16.1). The decision on which approach to use depends on a variety of factors; although patient tolerability is highest with the subclavian approach, it has also the highest incidence of acute complications.[2] The procedure should be performed under mild sedation, with ECG, blood pressure, and pulse oximetry monitoring.

Indications for the procedure are outlined in Table 16.1. The sole relative contraindication for the procedure is coagulopathy (INR > 1.8, PTT > 2× normal and/or platelet count < 50,000/mL).

Femoral Vein Approach

When this approach is used, the pacing catheter is advanced through the sheath for up to 15 cm, the balloon inflated, and the catheter is advanced into the RA under fluoroscopic guidance. Access to the RV usually follows the steps described in Chapter 10. If the RV has

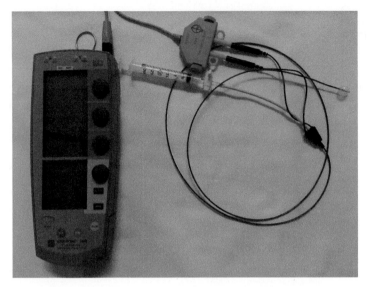

FIGURE 16.1   Temporary transvenous pacemaker equipment (Medtronic, Inc., Minneapolis, MN) is shown with a temporary transvenous balloon-tipped pacing catheter (C.R. Bard, Inc., Lowell, MA).

TABLE 16.1   Indications for temporary transvenous pacemaker placement.

1. Myocardial infarction complicated by:
   • New RBBB + LAFB, or LPFB
   • New LBBB + first-degree AV block
   • Alternating LBBB and RBBB
   • Mobitz type II second-degree AV block
   • Third-degree AV block
2. Hemodynamically significant bradycardia
3. Overdrive pacing for termination of certain types of arrhythmias (type I atrial flutter, AV-nodal reentry tachycardia)
4. Bridge to permanent pacing
5. Acute complete AV block secondary to sarcoidosis or myocarditis
6. Prophylactic, in anticipation of high degree AV block secondary to certain procedures (rotablation of RCA) in the catheterization laboratory

been reached by a pacing catheter creating a loop in the RA, the lead needs to be rotated to eliminate the loop, since this loop tends to point the tip of the lead upwards towards the RVOT. This placement should only be used if the catheter tip cannot be placed into the RV apex.

After crossing the tricuspid valve and entering the RV, the balloon is deflated. The lead should take a gentle arc through the tricuspid valve to be pointed inferiorly and the catheter turned clockwise, which will direct the tip of the catheter against the septum.

With proper positioning, there should be minimal movement of the lead in systole. The position of the lead is verified in RAO and LAO projections by fluoroscopy. Lead movement should be further tested by asking the patient to take several deep breaths and cough. The operator attaches the pacing catheter through the connecting cable to a temporary pacemaker and initiates pacing under fluoroscopy with 5 mA output at a rate 10–20 bpm faster than the intrinsic heart rate. If asystole or extreme bradycardia is present, pacing should be performed at a rate of 80 bpm.

If there are no captured beats, or there is diaphragmatic contraction accompanying pacing, the pacemaker lead should be repositioned. When capturing is achieved at 5 mA, the current is slowly decreased until loss of capture is observed. The lowest capturing current is defined as the capture threshold. Ideally, the capture threshold should be less than 1 mA. Pacing should be set at 2 to 3 times the threshold current to ensure a safety margin.

The next step is testing the sensing threshold, which is done by setting the pacing rate at 10–20 bpm less than the intrinsic rate with the pacemaker in its lowest millivolt recognition, and then gradually decreasing it until asynchronous pacing is identified. The pacemaker is then set at 50% of the margin of safety. After completion of the procedure, the operator secures the connections and the pacing catheter position and obtains a 12-lead surface ECG and chest x-ray. The patient should remain in bed in a supine position. A postprocedural chest x-ray is highly recommended even if fluoroscopy does not show an obvious pneumothorax.

Right Internal Jugular Vein Approach

When utilizing the jugular or subclavian vein approach, the pacing catheter is advanced through the 5-Fr sheath for up to 15 cm, the balloon is inflated, and the catheter moved into the RA. After crossing the tricuspid valve and entering the RV, the balloon is deflated, and the catheter tip is directed by clockwise rotation inferiorly towards the right ventricular apex. The proper position of the lead is suggested by its pointing to 4 to 5 o'clock, and to the edge of the cardiac silhouette. Subsequent steps are identical to the steps described for the femoral approach.

WHAT IF AN OPERATOR ENCOUNTERS ONE OF THE FOLLOWING PROBLEMS?

Chamber Perforation

RA or RV perforations (see also Chapter 10) during temporary pacemaker implantation with fluoroscopic and echocardiographic guidance are rare. If this complication occurs, it is frequently preceded by chest and shoulder pain and may be followed by vasovagal symptoms when blood enters the pericardium. These symptoms are accompanied by a sudden change in the pacing threshold, and/or a loss of pacing/sensing, and can be followed by the development of cardiac tamponade. Rarely, the temporary pacemaker wire may perforate the interventricular septum. This usually manifests itself by a sudden change of pacing threshold, and a change in the surface ECG from a characteristic LBBB to a RBBB, suggestive of LV pacing. Withdrawal of the lead and repositioning of its tip is necessary.

Pacemaker Failure

Failure to pace or sense is usually due to migration of the pacing wire, unless ventricular perforation has occurred or the pacemaker/generator is dysfunctional.

Arrhythmias

As the balloon-tipped lead enters the RA and passes into the RV, arrhythmias can occur, which in most cases are minor in nature and temporary in character (PACs and PVCs, RBBB). These abnormal beats are caused by the balloon-tipped catheter's contact with the endocardium, and can be easily terminated with a slight withdrawal of the lead. Sustained atrial or ventricular arrhythmias requiring treatment occur much less commonly, and primarily occur in patients with myocardial ischemia or myocardial infarction, pre-existing atrial or ventricular arrhythmias, or as a result of ineffective overdrive pacing. In such circumstances, the operator and the cath lab personnel follow the current ACLS guidelines to tackle the problem quickly and effectively.

In the presence of a complete LBBB, RBBB precipitated by the pacing wire results in complete heart block, which is usually short-lived. It is important for the cath lab personnel to be familiar with this problem and initiate temporary transcutaneous pacing if complete heart block persists. A prolonged episode of bradycardia accompanied by hypotension, nausea and sweating can be a manifestation of a vasovagal reaction, which may be triggered by right heart catheterization, especially in anxious patients with some element of volume depletion. To treat this generally benign complication, the operator initiates rapid volume administration combined with transvenous pacing and elevation of lower extremities. On rare occasions, if hypotension is not responding to the above measures, intravenous inotropic agents can be used.

References

1. Goldberger J, Kruse J, Ehlert FA, Kadish A. Temporary transvenous pacemaker placement: what criteria constitute an adequate pacing site? *Am Heart J.* 1993;126(2):488-493.
2. Cooper JP, Swanton RH. Complications of transvenous temporary pacemaker insertion. *Br J Hosp Med.* 1995;53(4):155-161.

CHAPTER 17

Post-Cardiac Catheterization Care

"It's never over till it's over."

—American Proverb

Documentation of the Procedure

Proper, early post-cardiac catheterization care with continuous vital signs, O_2 saturation, and ECG monitoring is extremely important for the safety of the patient, since even the best precatheterization evaluation and planning and a perfectly performed procedure can be ruined with careless postcatheterization care. After completion of the procedure, the operator reviews the obtained data and writes the final catheterization report.[1] The final catheterization procedure report is to be organized into 3 primary sections, containing section-specific content (Table 17.1). The first section is a brief (single page), easily understood, focused summary of the salient points that is directed to the clinical community. All clinicians should not need to look further than this first section of the report to ascertain the procedures performed, diagnostic findings, and recommendations.

The second section is focused on images of the observed anatomy, findings, and results. Captured images (with or without annotations) can be included in this section. Finally, the third section includes the details of the procedure. This includes administrative data, the preprocedure history, most of the procedural detail, free-text descriptions of technical details, and other content relevant to the final procedure report.

TABLE 17.1   Important elements of the physician's final cardiac catheterization report.

- Focused summary of the salient points directed to the clinical community
- Images
- Details of the procedure

Detailed samples of organization of the structured catheterization procedure report and diagnostic procedure report content are outlined in ACC/AHA/SCAI 2014 Health Policy Statement on Structured Reporting for the Cardiac Catheterization Laboratory: A Report of the American College of Cardiology Clinical Quality Committee.[1]

It is important to contact the referring physician and discuss the findings of the procedure. Based on this discussion, any required early postprocedural changes in the patient's care will be implemented. The operator explains the final findings to the patient in layman's terms, discusses potential options for therapy, and provides either printed pictures or a digital copy of the coronary angiography for the patient's personal medical file. While the patient is in the cardiac catheterization observation unit, the nursing staff needs to be vigilant for early detection of symptoms and signs indicative of possible postprocedural complications, since even mild changes in a patient's condition after cardiac catheterization may be a harbinger of impending hemodynamic compromise. A focal baseline neurologic examination conducted by the operator postprocedure is highly recommended, with particular attention toward any change from the preprocedural examination.

If the patient's condition remains stable, and the access site has been checked, the operator instructs the patient to follow certain rules (Table 17.2). Compliance with these rules assists the normal

TABLE 17.2   Temporary restrictions after cardiac catheterization.

Radial and Brachial Approaches:
- No strenuous activity for 48 hours involving the arms
- Dressing removed in 24 hours
- Area of access site should be kept dry and clean

Femoral Approach:
- No strenuous activity for 36–48 hours, including driving
- Dressing removed in 24 hours
- Shower in 24 hours
- No bathing or swimming until the access site is completely healed

TABLE 17.3   Possible late complications after cardiac catheterization.

- Local infection/inflammation: redness, local swelling, discharge, pain, and increase in temperature
- Bleeding or slow oozing
- Ischemic limb: numbness, pain, loss of color, absence of distal pulses, cold limb, absence of appropriate limb function
- Pseudoaneurysm: local swelling with or without accompanying pain

healing process of the access site. No other restrictions or routine laboratory checks apply unless the patient's condition has changed. The patient is informed about signs of possible late complications (Table 17.3) of cardiac catheterization and detailed information is provided about how to act if such conditions occur. After all these steps are completed and the patient's appropriate follow-up is arranged, the patient can be discharged from the cardiac catheterization observation unit.

Vascular Access Site Closure

MANUAL COMPRESSION

Despite its obvious limitations, such as patient discomfort, prolonged bedrest, and interruption of anticoagulation, manual compression is still considered the gold standard of achieving hemostasis post arterial sheath removal, since none of the closure devices in randomized trials were able to show a significant reduction in vascular complications.[2-5] The process of removing the arterial sheath and achieving local hemostasis by digital pressure is relatively simple but requires adherence to certain rules. Prior to removing a sheath, the operator should make sure that the patient is positioned correctly. In case of femoral sheath removal, the patient should be in a recumbent position close to the edge of the bed, with the bed height adjusted so that the pressure vector applied by the operator's fingers is oriented vertically to the femoral arterial access site. In cases of brachial or radial arterial sheath removal, the position of the patient and operator follows common sense of comfort for both. It is important for the operator that the patient's vital signs can be seen on the monitor, intravenous access is working properly, 1 mg atropine solution is available, sterile 4 × 4 pads, alcohol swabs, suture removal kit, 10-mL syringe, and a pair of sterile gloves are on the table. The procedure is briefly explained to the patient, distal pulses are checked, the syringe is connected to the side port of the sheath, and 3–4 mL of blood is aspirated. The skin around the sheath entrance is cleaned by alcohol swabs and then a couple of 4×4 pads are placed just below the hub of the sheath. The operator positions the left hand (in case of right femoral artery access) and palpates the arterial pulse about 1–1.5 cm above the skin entrance of the sheath (the cutaneous landmark of the needle entry into the artery is located about 0.5–1 cm superior, due to the cranial direction of the entry needle during arterial access). The index finger is then placed on the pulse about 0.5–1 cm below the skin entrance of the sheath, so that the skin nick remains visible at all times for applied pressure control and detection of any bleeding due to insufficient or malpositioned manual pressure. After positioning the operator's fingers on the pulse as described, the patient is notified that pressure will be applied at the site and asked to breathe normally and to relax. With the index finger slowly but steadily applying occlusive pressure to the distal artery, the sheath is withdrawn by the hub using the other hand. The operator allows a few seconds of bleeding before firm, direct, occlusive pressure is applied with the fingers at the proximal point and the pressure on the distal point applied by the index finger is released. As soon as complete occlusion of the proximal vessel is achieved, the operator gradually decreases the pressure applied by the middle and ring fingers until able to feel a femoral pulsation, which is suggestive of partial resumption of antegrade flow. Firm pressure is maintained for 3–5 minutes, after which digital pressure is gradually reduced over the next 10–15 minutes (5–10 minutes with 4-Fr sheath) with constant observation of the site. The operator uses the other hand to periodically palpate and check the area around the access site to prevent and/or detect early hematoma formation deep below the skin surface.

Once compression is released, the site is observed for a full minute, and distal pulses are checked. If bleeding resumes, another 10–15 minutes of pressure is applied. Otherwise, the access site is covered with a translucent, sterile adhesive plastic cover, and the patient is advised to remain in a horizontal position with head relaxed on the pillow for 1 hour with frequent site checks. If there are no signs of bleeding, the patient is placed at a 30- to 45-degree upright angle with the accessed leg straight for the remainder of the observation (total observation time: 4-Fr sheath, 2 hours; 5-Fr sheath, 3 hours, 6-Fr sheath, 4 hours). No pressure dressing, such as a sand bag, is recommended for the access site. A sand bag obstructs venous flow and does not decrease the rate of arterial bleeding; it obscures the vision of the operator, which can lead to a large amount of blood loss going unnoticed. After the observation period is completed, a physician checks the site for presence of a hematoma, active oozing, and new bruits and rechecks the distal pulses, leg motion, and sensitivity. The patient is asked to cough gently while the area is monitored. The patient is allowed to get up in the presence of a nurse and ambulate only after the above check is completed. The site is reinspected prior to discharge.

When dealing with manual compression of the access site in artificial ileo- or aorto-femoral grafts, the operator needs to exercise extra caution in order to not compress the graft completely, but rather apply minimal sufficient pressure to prevent bleeding from the site for 15–20 minutes. Occlusive pressure to the graft may lead to graft thrombosis and should be avoided.

Risk factors for recurrent bleeding which may cause the operator to modify duration of manual compression and observation include:

- Severe atherosclerosis and calcification of the access vessel (loss of elasticity)
- High blood pressure
- Chronic renal insufficiency (dysfunctional platelets)
- Obesity
- Severe aortic regurgitation (wide pulse pressure)
- Coagulopathy
- Thrombocytopenia
- Continuous $Gp_{IIb/IIIa}$ receptor antagonist infusion

If periprocedural intravenous unfractionated heparin has been used, activated clotting time (ACT) should be checked prior to femoral arterial sheath removal. The femoral sheath can be safely removed if ACT is less than 180 seconds. In case of left and right cardiac catheterization, the femoral venous sheath should be flushed periodically while the arterial site compression is maintained, and removed after arterial hemostasis has been achieved.

VASCULAR CLOSURE DEVICES

The SyvekPatch (Marine Polymer Technologies, Danvers, MA, USA)[6] and V+Pad (Angiotech Pharmaceuticals Inc., Vancouver, BC, Canada) are small pads frequently used to promote clot formation and stabilization at the femoral arterial access site.[7,8] After palpating the proximal pulse and prior to sheath removal, the operator positions and fixes the edge of the patch under the middle finger so that the body of the patch covers the hub of the sheath. When the sheath is removed, backflow of blood wets the patch prior to proximal occlusive pressure being applied to the artery. Subsequently, the index finger of the same hand moves from the distal position to directly over the patch, where pressure is applied for 10–15 minutes until stable hemostasis is obtained. Once hemostasis has been confirmed, the dry adhesive translucent dressing is applied over the patch. The rest of the steps are identical to the steps described for manual compression. Within 24 hours, the water-moistened patch can be gently peeled off by the patient. The major advantages of these patches are absence of foreign body deployment into the access site; availability of the same access site for immediate use if needed; and ability to shorten the observation period and allow early ambulation (2 hours) of a patient. It is not recommended to use SyvekPatch or V+Pad for patients with artificial ileo-femoral or aorto-femoral grafts.

C-Arm Clamp

There are no advantages of using a C-arm clamp versus manual compression except for freeing up the staff to perform other duties in a busy catheterization laboratory, especially when prolonged manual compression of the site is required (Figure 17.1). Limitations include inability to regulate pressure easily and use in emergency. The C-arm clamp is a simple device which has a flat base and a reverse "L"-type arm attached to the base at 90 degrees. The distal tip of the device is attached to a disposable plastic disk. In order to correctly place the C-arm clamp, a patient is placed in recumbent position close to the edge of the bed where the hip of the patient rests directly over the flat base of the clamp. In the proper position, the movable transparent plastic disk, which plays the role of the pressure applicator for the C-arm clamp, should be projecting directly over the access site, slightly higher than the hub of the sheath, which has been moved back for about 1–1.5 cm, and direct moderate pressure is applied to the access site from the down motion of the plastic disk. The sheath is removed and occlusive pressure applied. The initial occlusive pressure is gradually released over 15 minutes without permitting bleeding from the puncture site and to allow distal blood circulation with close monitoring of distal pulses. The operator periodically palpates and checks the area

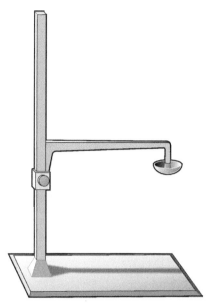

FIGURE 17.1   A C-clamp may be used to provide arterial compression.

around the access site to prevent and/or detect early hematoma formation deep below the skin surface.

Once arterial compression is completed, subsequent care of the access site is routine as described for manual compression. It is contraindicated to use a C-clamp for patients with artificial ileo-femoral or aorto-femoral grafts.

FemoStop

The advantages of a FemoStop (FemoStop plus, RADI Medical Systems AB, Uppsala, Sweden) over the C-arm clamp include easily controlled pressure monitoring, the ability to use it in acute situations, and preserved transportability of the patient (Figure 17.2). The FemoStop is a pneumatic pressure device used to obtain hemostasis after vascular sheath removal.[7] It can be also effectively used to control compressible arterial pseudoaneurysms at the access site. The FemoStop device consists of a plastic arch, to which an air-cushioned, transparent dome is attached with a polyester belt, and a reusable pump. In order to correctly place the FemoStop device, the patient should be placed in a recumbent position where the hips and lower back of the patient rest directly over the polyester belt threaded into the fastening device of the plastic arch of the FemoStop.

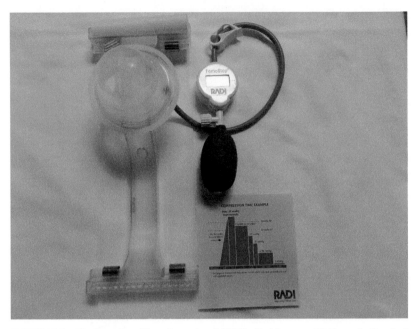

FIGURE 17.2   The FemoStop (FemoStop plus, RADI Medical Systems AB, Uppsala, Sweden) is a pneumatic pressure device that offers an alternative to a C-clamp.

In the proper position, the movable, air-cushioned, transparent plastic disk/dome, which functions as a pressure applicator of the FemoStop device, should be projecting directly over the access site slightly above the hub of the sheath, which should be withdrawn about 1–1.5 cm. Once the system is ready for use, the operator peels off the protective lid, exposing the sterile surface of the dome, which has been already connected to a reusable precision-controlled manometer pump through the stopcock. Direct, moderate pressure is "dialed in" by pumping air into the dome as it sits over the site; the sheath is removed, and additional occlusive pressure is "dialed in." The initial occlusive pressure is then gradually released over the next 3 minutes without permitting bleeding from the puncture site and allowing distal blood circulation with close monitoring of the quality of the distal pulses. The operator keeps the dome pressure above the patient's diastolic pressure for the next 15 minutes, after which the dome pressure is gradually reduced to 40 mm Hg over the next 4 minutes and then further reduced to around 30 mm Hg. The duration of compression depends on several factors including sheath size and anticoagulation status. The operator periodically palpates and checks the area around the access site to prevent and/

or detect early hematoma formation. Once arterial compression is completed, subsequent care of the access site is routine as described for manual compression. In case of a femoral venous sheath, the dome is inflated to 20–30 mm Hg and the sheath is removed. To minimize the risk of AV fistula formation, venous hemostasis should be achieved prior to removal of the arterial sheath.

Both C-arm clamp and FemoStop mechanical compression devices have contraindications (Table 17.4) and adverse effects (Table 17.5) that may occur. Hence, the physician should carefully weigh the risks and benefits prior to application of these devices in each individual case.

Obtaining Hemostasis of the Radial Arteriotomy Site

PREPARATION

Upon completion of cardiac catheterization, the operator withdraws blood and flushes the radial sheath with heparinized saline.[8] The area of the wrist surrounding the arteriotomy site and the

TABLE 17.4   **Possible adverse effects.**

- Tissue necrosis
- Blistering of skin/skin abrasions
- Compression injuries to nerves
- Femoral artery and/or vein thrombosis
- Embolization
- Bleeding or hematoma
- Arteriovenous fistula or pseudoaneurysm formation
- Acute distension or rupture of a pseudoaneurysm during ultrasound-guided compression repair

TABLE 17.5   **Contraindications.**

- Severe peripheral vascular disease due to risk of thrombosis
- Critical limb ischemia
- Overlying skin necrosis and/or infection
- Arterial injuries above or near the inguinal ligament
- Inability to adequately compress the site
- Femoral artery graft or stent, or vein graft due to risk of damage and thrombosis
- Ultrasound-guided compression repair of infected femoral pseudoaneurysms
- Patients not suitable for compression of their femoral artery due to severe leg edema, femoral nerve compression, or arterial obstruction

radial sheath are cleaned using a topical bacteriostatic agent such as chlorhexidine. The radial sheath is withdrawn for 2–3 cm. If any resistance is felt, or if the patient complains of significant pain or discomfort, the operator should consider injecting local/subcutaneous 1% lidocaine, and an intra-arterial vasodilator such as verapamil, or nitroglycerin, to ease vasospasm prior to reattempting partial sheath withdrawal.

WRISTBAND AND SHEATH REMOVAL

The operator aligns the green marker located in the center of the compression wristband just proximal to where the sheath enters the arteriotomy site. The Velcro strap is fixed around the wrist (Figure 17.3). Approximately 15 mL of air volume is aspirated into the syringe included in the kit. This prefilled syringe is attached to the compression balloon side port of the wristband. With the syringe in one hand, air is injected into the compression balloon in

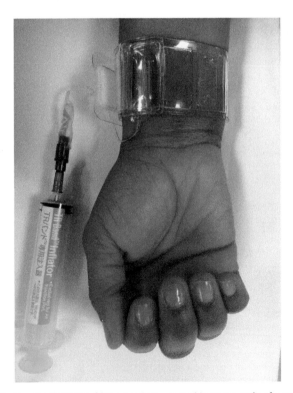

FIGURE 17.3   Terumo Wrist Band (Terumo Corp., Japan) is an example of a compression wristband.

order to inflate the wristband around the arteriotomy site, while pulling back and completely removing the arterial sheath with the other hand.

The arteriotomy site is closely monitored through the transparent wristband to confirm hemostasis, possibly injecting more air volume if needed (the maximum air volume that can be injected is 18 mL). Air is gradually withdrawn 1 mL at a time, looking for a blush of blood from the arteriotomy site. Once blush is observed, withdrawal is stopped, and the balloon is reinflated with additional 3 cc of air. This ensures adequate compression pressure for hemostasis but prevents excessive compression of the radial artery. The syringe is disconnected and the final amount of air injected into the wristband is recorded.

Confirming Patent Circulation of the Hand

The patent radial arterial circulation distal to the wristband should be confirmed either by palpation of the radial artery just distal to the wristband or by monitoring the amplitude and morphology of the pulse oximetry wave form with the sensor placed on one of the 3 lateral digits of the hand.

MYNX GRIP CLOSURE DEVICE

The Mynx Grip (AccessClosure, Mountain View, CA) is a balloon-catheter sealing device that uses polyethylene glycol, a water-soluble, bioinert, nonthrombogenic polymer, as a sealant. When delivered to the tissue tract, the freeze-dried polyethylene glycol sealant instantly absorbs blood and fluids, swells approximately 3–4 times its size, and provides immediate hemostasis (Figure 17.4). This device can be used for 5-Fr to 7-Fr sheaths, and the only major contraindication for its use is a high-access needle stick. Within 30 days from deployment, the sealant dissolves completely. Predeployment femoral angiography is required.

The process of deployment starts with gentle insertion of the device by the operator through the existing introducer sheath and the subsequent inflation of a small, semicompliant balloon inside the artery. The operator gently moves the balloon back until it anchors the arteriotomy site from the inner wall of the artery; the sealant is then delivered and unsleeved. Moderate pressure is applied for 30 seconds, with subsequent 90 seconds dwell time, followed by deflation of the balloon and removal of the device. Manual compression is applied for 1 minute until complete hemostasis is achieved.

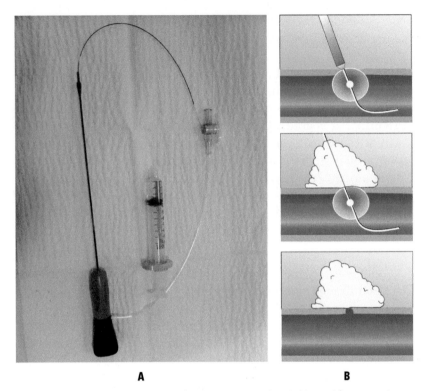

A   B

FIGURE 17.4   The Mynx Grip (AccessClosure, Mountain View, CA) is used for access site closure. **Panel A**: The Mynx Grip device is shown. **Panel B**: Steps for closure of access site are shown.

Once manual compression is completed, the site is observed for a full 1 minute, reexamined for presence of subcutaneous hematoma, and distal pulses are checked. Occasionally, when dealing with a severely calcified vessel, there is risk of puncturing the semicompliant balloon with the sharp edge of vessel wall calcium; this will lead to a failure to deploy the device and will require manual compression. Some operators would prefer to save the arterial access site by running a 0.025-inch guidewire parallel to the Mynx device, and if an accidental rupture of the balloon occurs, preserve the access and reattempt to deploy the closure device. Otherwise, if no major problem occurs, the guidewire can be removed. Subsequent care of the access site is routine as described for manual compression. The patient can be discharged home after 2 hours from the point of successful deployment of the device. There are no restrictions to use the same site for vascular access immediately if needed.

ANGIO-SEAL STS PLUS CLOSURE DEVICE

The Angio-Seal STS Plus (St. Jude Medical, St. Paul, MN) is an anchor-based, collagen-plug closure device that uses a flat rectangular anchor plate abutting the artery from inside, a purified collagen plug deployed to the arterial outside surface, and a suture material tethering the 2 elements together, producing virtually immediate hemostasis, usually without manual compression (Figure 17.5). All 3 foreign bodies deployed into the access site are resorbed in 30 to 90 days.

The process of deployment starts with obtaining a femoral artery angiogram in RAO projection followed by verification that no contraindications (Table 17.6) to device placement exist and reviewing of the precautions in device placement (Table 17.7). These steps are followed by the introduction of the 0.035-inch guidewire through the existing 6-Fr or 7-Fr arterial sheath, sheath removal over the guidewire, and application of occlusive digital pressure about 1–1.5 cm above the access site.

A construct composed of a device sheath of the same French size with a dilator/arteriotomy locator inserted through it is assembled, flushed, gently placed over the guidewire into the vessel lumen, and advanced until blood return is observed through the proximal side hole of the arteriotomy locator. Slight backward movement of the

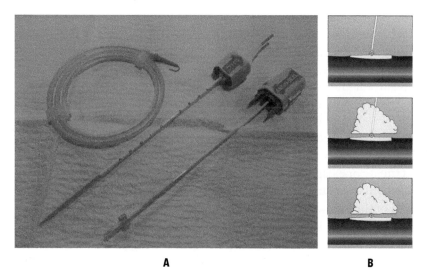

A   **B**

FIGURE 17.5   The Angio-Seal STS Plus (St. Jude Medical, Minnetonka, MN) is an alternate closure device. **Panel A**: The Angio-Seal STS Plus device is shown. **Panel B**: Steps for closure of access site are shown.

TABLE 17.6   Contraindications to device placement.

- Bacterial contamination of the procedure sheath or surrounding tissues
- A sheath that has been placed through the superficial femoral artery and into the profunda femoris may result in collagen deposition into the superficial femoral artery and may reduce blood flow through the vessel leading to symptoms of distal arterial insufficiency
- A puncture site at or distal to the bifurcation of the superficial femoral and profunda femoris arteries may result in (1) the anchor catching on the bifurcation or being positioned incorrectly, and/or (2) collagen deposition into the vessel. These events may reduce blood flow through the vessel leading to symptoms of distal arterial insufficiency
- A puncture site proximal to the inguinal ligament may result in retroperitoneal hematoma

TABLE 17.7   Precautions in device placement.

- Patients undergoing an interventional procedure who are being treated with warfarin
- Patients who have known allergies to beef products, collagen and/or collagen products, or polyglycolic or polylactic acid polymers
- Patients with preexisting autoimmune disease
- Patients undergoing therapeutic thrombolysis
- Patient's blood vessel punctured through a vascular graft
- Patients with uncontrolled hypertension (> 180 mm Hg systolic BP)
- Patients with a bleeding disorder, including thrombocytopenia (< 75,000 platelets/mL)
- Pediatric patients or others with small femoral artery size (< 4 mm in diameter); small femoral artery size may prevent the ANGIO-SEAL anchor from proper deployment
- Women who are pregnant or lactating

entire construct, performed by the operator, leads to the stoppage of blood return (indicates that the distal locator holes of the device have exited the artery). This step is followed again by advancement and reappearance of blood return through the side hole. At this point, the operator fixes the position of the sheath and removes the arteriotomy locator and wire by flexing the arteriotomy locator upward at the sheath hub. This is followed by the anchor delivery to the vessel through the designated sheath until the sheath cap and the device sleeve snap together. Next the operator holds the sheath and slowly and carefully pulls the device cap back into the full rear-locked position with the other hand. Some resistance is usually felt as the device cap and sleeve snap lock. The operator withdraws the device until the anchor catches correctly and abuts to the inside wall of the vessel. While maintaining tension on the suture, the collagen plug is pushed down into the skin track onto the outside of the arterial wall. With the tamper tube, the suture tightens, a knot forms, and hemostasis is achieved within the next several seconds.

The suture is trimmed below skin level by applying mild pressure on the tissue around the site. If oozing persists, 2–3 minutes of nonocclusive manual pressure is applied on the site. The operator should exercise caution and not apply too much tension when pull-ing, since this may cause the disc to pull out of the vessel. When hemostasis has been achieved, the access site is cleaned with an antiseptic solution and covered with a translucent, sterile, adhe-sive plastic dressing. The patient remains in a horizontal position with head relaxed on the pillow for 5–10 minutes, during which the site gets checked frequently. If there are no signs of bleeding, the patient is placed at a 45-degree upright angle with the leg remain-ing straight for an additional 20–25 minutes. After this period, the patient is permitted to bend his/her leg. Subsequent care of the access site is routine as described for manual compression. Patients can be discharged home after 2 hours from the point of successful deployment of the device. It is generally recommended not to use the same site for vascular access for the next 90 days.

STARCLOSE DEVICE

The StarClose device (Abbott Vascular, Redwood, CA) is a nitinol clip-based closure device that, upon deployment, leads to active approximation of the vessel wall, with the deposition of the perma-nent device on the surface of the femoral artery penetrating only to the arterial media, and avoiding placement of a collagen plug or suture material in the tissue tract (Figure 17.6). The process of

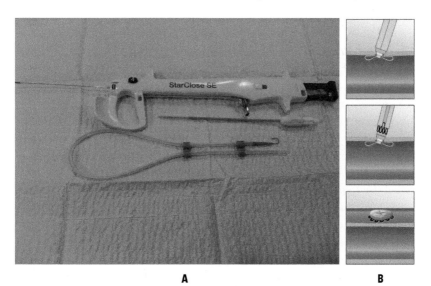

A   **B**

FIGURE 17.6   The StarClose device (Abbott Vascular, Redwood, CA) is used for access site closure. **Panel A**: The device and associated attachments are shown. **Panel B**: The steps used to achieve access site closure are shown.

deployment starts with exchanging an existing sheath over the wire with a specifically designed sheath from the closure kit, usually 6- or 7-Fr in diameter. After positioning the wire, the original sheath is removed; the wire is kept in place to prevent loss of access. If the tissue tract has not been prepared before positioning the original sheath, the operator dilates the tract with the forceps. Then the sheath from the StarClose kit is placed over the wire into the vessel. Subsequently, the operator runs the tip of the StarClose device through the sheath, and the sheath is moved slightly back so that the hub is positioned about 0.5 cm from the skin surface. This will provide a space to support the sheath with the index and middle fingers of the operator, once the other hand has advanced the device until it clicks with the hub of the sheath. When this step is completed, the operator, by pushing button #2 of the device, opens the umbrella-type structure at the distal tip of the StarClose device and slowly retrieves the device–sheath construct until the distal tip/umbrella of the device is anchored at the vessel wall. At this point, the device is fixed in position with the left hand, and by advancing button #3 on the StarClose device, the sheath gets split all the way to its distal end. Then, the operator changes the angle of the deployment device to approximately 70–80 degrees, makes sure that the distal tip/umbrella of the device is still resting on the inner surface of the vessel wall, and pushes button #4, delivering the nitinol clip to the vessel wall.

After the ring is deployed, the StarClose delivery system is slowly withdrawn, and if no resistance is met, removed. This is followed by mild manual compression to the site for one minute, after which the site is checked for bleeding. If significant resistance occurs while removing the delivery system, button #3 should be released by using the sheath introducer tip to apply pressure sequentially to the 2 small releasing points/holes; after the pressure is withdrawn, the system usually is removed without a problem. If no bleeding is noted, the patient is asked to give a strong cough and bend the leg on the access site, and if again no bleeding is noted, the device has been successfully deployed. When hemostasis has been achieved, the access site is cleaned with an antiseptic solution and is covered with a translucent sterile adhesive plastic dressing. The patient remains in a horizontal position with the head relaxed on the pillow for 5 minutes, and the site is checked. If there are no signs of bleeding, the patient is placed at a 45-degree upright angle in the bed with no major restriction of bending the leg. After an additional hour the site should be checked.

Subsequent care of the access site is routine as described for manual compression. Patients can be discharged home after one hour from the point of successful deployment of the device. There are generally no restrictions to use the same site for vascular access immediately if needed.

WHAT IF AN OPERATOR ENCOUNTERS ONE OF THE FOLLOWING PROBLEMS?

Access Site Bleeding Occurs After the Cardiac Catheterization Procedure

Arterial access site bleeding occurs more often than venous access site bleeding for obvious reasons, and it requires a faster, more aggressive response from the operator and observation unit nurses. Immediate manual compression of the access site to establish control over the bleeding is the initial step. This will control bleeding unless the access site is high above the inguinal ligament, where the effectiveness of manual compression is decreased significantly.

There are certain factors associated with increased risk of access site bleeding (Table 17.8), and patients with these risk factors should be carefully monitored.

If the access site is located below the inguinal ligament, a local soft-tissue hematoma may form. It can lead to a significant drop in the patient's hemoglobin concentration, hypotension, compensatory tachycardia, or hemodynamic instability, requiring urgent blood transfusion. Such a development is not frequently found in a fully awake patient, since in most cases focal discomfort and pain accompanying hematoma formation lead to early detection of bleeding at the access site. When bleeding from the access site is controlled and the patient's hemodynamics are stabilized, the visible borders of the hematoma are demarcated and its size estimated. If a moderate- or large-size hematoma has formed, the operator

TABLE 17.8 Risk factors for bleeding at the access site.

- Female patient
- Hypertension
- Obesity
- Large-diameter sheath
- Low body weight
- Old age
- Anticoagulant or thrombolytic on board
- Prolonged indwelling sheath
- End-stage renal disease

continues to apply further diffuse, compressive pressure with the palm of the hand in order to transform a hard hematoma into a soft one by moving the focal collection of blood into a broad area of nearby subcutaneous soft tissue of the upper thigh. This process could be very painful for a patient, so appropriate short-acting analgesics are often needed. Large hematomas can compress the femoral vein and predispose the patient towards developing deep vein thrombosis.[9] In very large hematomas, surgical consultation may be appropriate, although surgical repair of hematomas is generally not required. A Doppler ultrasound revealing the absence of blood flow from the arterial vessel towards the hematoma differentiates it from pseudoaneurysm. A CT scan may be required to assess the extent of a hematoma and to rule out retroperitoneal bleeding.

If the arterial access site is located above the inguinal ligament and above the inferior epigastric artery, the internal bleeding might not be diagnosed in timely fashion and can lead to retroperitoneal hematoma formation, followed by hemodynamic instability and potential death of the patient. In general, patients with this complication present with new, unexplained tachycardia and hypotension accompanied by ipsilateral flank or back pain, flank ecchymosis, and femoral neuropathy. When the above signs or symptoms occur, hemoglobin/hematocrit levels should be obtained immediately, fluid resuscitation initiated, patient's blood typed and screened, anticoagulant and antiplatelet therapy stopped, and a noncontrast abdomen and pelvis CT scan performed. If the latter is not available, abdominal and pelvic ultrasound can be used to establish the diagnosis. When the diagnosis of retroperitoneal hematoma is proven, volume resuscitation, with or without blood transfusion, should be the cornerstone of therapy. The decision on reversal of anticoagulation and platelet transfusion should be made by the physician on a case-by-case basis. Surgical correction of this complication is rarely required. Occasionally, if surgical support is not available and the patient's hemodynamics cannot be stabilized with blood and fluid transfusions/infusions, some operators may proceed with emergent angiography from the contralateral femoral access site to localize the bleeding site. Once the bleeding site has been identified, it can be controlled by inflating an appropriate size angioplasty balloon or by placing a covered stent.[10]

Pseudoaneurysm

In up to 1% of all diagnostic left heart catheterizations, a pseudoaneurysm can form at the arterial access site.[11] This complication is characterized by disruption in all 3 major layers of the arterial wall with formation of the contained hematoma. Patients usually present somewhat later in the postcatheterization period, and symptoms are frequently described as sudden sharp pain at the access site followed by local swelling, frequently preceded by some physical activity accompanied by strain.

In general, pseudoaneurysms occur in the presence of inadequate sealing of the arterial puncture site. Patients with higher risk of developing this complication are older, female, obese, or have diabetes. Other risk factors include lower arterial access at the superficial femoral or profunda femoris artery and a very brief period of manual compression after the sheath removal if a closure device is not used. On the postcatheterization examination, a pseudoaneurysm should be suspected if there is local pain and/or a pulsating and enlarging mass accompanied by limb weakness and paresthesia. A systolic bruit can be heard when auscultating the enlarged and pulsating mass. The diagnosis of a pseudoaneurysm can best be confirmed by color flow Doppler ultrasound. Small pseudoaneurysms (< 2 cm) tend to clot off spontaneously. In contrast, larger pseudoaneurysms are predisposed to spontaneous rupture. Most pseudoaneurysms can be treated with direct, ultrasound-guided compression or with ultrasound-guided local injection of thrombin or biodegradable collagen into the pseudoaneurysm cavity. Ultrasound-guided direct compression, although effective, is uncomfortable for the patient. It is also time-consuming (average compression time around 30–45 minutes) and labor-intensive. The failure rate varies and can be as high as 15%, especially in patients on concomitant anticoagulation therapy, with obesity, or large pseudoaneurysms. Ultrasound-guided thrombin injection (500–1000 U) can be performed with or without angioplasty balloon protection of the true vessel lumen. If an angioplasty balloon is not used, the operator needs to direct the needle tip away from the neck of the pseudoaneurysm in order to avoid distal thrombin embolization. Aliquots of 0.2 mL (1000 U/mL) are injected and visualized with color Doppler until no flow is observed, which usually occurs within seconds. On the other hand, when the angioplasty balloon is used, the contralateral site is accessed, a sheath is placed, and a guidewire is run and directed with the help of a JR or IMA catheter around the iliac bifurcation distally towards the affected femoral site. Subsequently, the peripheral angioplasty balloon, sized 1:1 to the diameter of the reference vessel, is deployed across the origin of the pseudoaneurysm. A small amount of thrombin is then percutaneously injected into the sac with no risk for distal emboli-zation. Covered stents and coil embolization can also be used suc-cessfully to treat pseudoaneurysms. Vascular surgery is standard of care in cases when large pseudoaneurysms develop at the site of vascular anastomosis, or with infected pseudoaneurysms.

Arteriovenous Fistula Formation

Arteriovenous fistulas form when the access needle punctures 2 vascular structures, artery and vein, while the operator advances the needle during vascular access. The most frequent cause is either an anatomical position of the vein, a low stick, or incorrect direc-tion of the access needle. This fistulous tract may remain open after the completion of the cardiac catheterization procedure and sheath removal. During the postcatheterization examination of the access site, the operator should meticulously auscultate the area and sus-pect arteriovenous fistula if there is continuous to-and-fro bruit heard on auscultation. In extreme cases a pulsatile mass with or without continuous enlargement accompanied by diminished distal pulses can be noticed on examination. The diagnosis of, arteriove-nous fistula can be confirmed by color flow Doppler ultrasound. Smaller fistulas are not hemodynamically significant and close spontaneously or with ultrasound-guided compression. Larger fis-tulas may cause symptoms and need to be closed by vascular sur-gery. Percutaneous closure of fistulas has been performed in rare cases by using covered stents and coil embolization.[12]

Neuropathy

Femoral neuropathy occurs rarely, and most of the time is related to an accidental needle stick or local anesthetic injection. Another frequent cause is related to prolonged horizontal immobilization of patients with severe osteochondrosis of the lumbar spine (L2–L4 vertebrae). Changing the position from supine to sitting takes care of the latter problem within a short period of time (hours). Occasionally, femoral neuropathy develops as a result of local com-pression secondary to retroperitoneal or inguinal hematomas, which by their nature could be vascular access complications. The motor component of the femoral nerve innervates the muscles responsible for hip flexion and knee extension; when compressed, symptoms are characterized by the patient's inability to ambulate or patient complaint of leg or knee "giving up" or "buckling." This problem can go completely unnoticed when the patient remains in a supine position, revealing itself only if specifically checked (e.g., physical examination noting decreased strength of the quadriceps muscle and diminished patellar reflex) or when the patient attempts to stand up. The observation unit nurse caring for the patient should instruct the patient to get up slowly and make sure that there is support for the patient if his/her leg becomes weak. In addition, if the patient develops difficulty bending the hip, a retroperitoneal hematoma compressing the femoral nerve should be suspected as a cause, since the motor branch of the femoral nerve for the iliopsoas muscle (controls flexion of the hip) comes off above the inguinal ligament.

In general, after appropriate imaging studies (inguinal ultrasound, abdominal/pelvis CT scan), the therapeutic approach is conservative, but surgical decompression of the nerve sometimes may be required secondary to large inguinal or retroperitoneal hematomas.

It should also be noted that the sensory branch of the femoral nerve innervates the skin of the medial thigh and the anterior and medial aspects of the calf. Injection of a local anesthetic or compression of this branch can lead to numbness and paresthesia in these skin zones, which in case of direct injection of the anesthetic could last up to several weeks, occasionally months.

Local hematoma formation is the most frequent cause of medial brachial fascial compartment syndrome when the brachial artery approach is utilized for cardiac catheterization. The median and ulnar nerves are most frequently affected. Initial symptoms of medial brachial fascial compartment syndrome, such as unilateral pain and paresthesia, may be followed by progressive weakness of the thenar aspect of the hand and occur several days after the procedure. Distal pulses usually remain normal. Urgent surgical decompression is indicated.

Limb Ischemia

Arterial thrombosis at the access site can occur and may lead to limb ischemia.[12] Iatrogenic dissection, local spasm (especially in the presence of a large-diameter sheath), severe peripheral vascular disease, diabetes, severe systolic dysfunction, and hypercoagulable state can lead to local thrombosis and limb ischemia.

Classical signs and symptoms of an acute limb ischemia consist of the five "Ps": pain, pallor, pulseless, paresthesia, and polar cold. The diagnosis may be confirmed by Doppler ultrasound. Patients with acute symptomatic limb ischemia that develops postcatheterization should undergo angiography to characterize the anatomic basis for the ischemia. Treatment options vary depending on the findings and could include percutaneous approaches (balloon angioplasty and stenting, with or without a selective infusion of thrombolytic therapy or catheter thrombectomy) or surgical approaches (thrombectomy and repair). Time of intervention on the ischemic limb is crucial, since delay of more than 6 hours may lead to extensive muscle necrosis followed by reperfusion injury when blood flow is restored.

Embolism

Atheroembolism is more frequent among patients with known severe atherosclerosis of the aorta and its main branches. It can potentially affect any organ, but in clinical practice, atheroembolic renal dysfunction occurring 7 days after the cardiac catheterization procedure is of particular significance, since it may persist and progress over several months in some cases. The exact mechanism of this phenomenon is not well established; it involves local obstruction of small (100–300 µm in diameter) vessels by atherosclerotic debris and a severe inflammatory response accompanied by elevation of the erythrocyte sedimentation rate, decreased complement level, eosinophiluria, and significant (> 3%) eosinophilia. In addition, clinical signs of systemic embolism, such as Hollenhorst plaques, limb pain, livedo reticularis, petechiae, digital infarctions, and splinter hemorrhages with preserved distal pulses can be observed.[13]

Management of atheroembolic renal dysfunction is mostly supportive, and in severe renal dysfunction, hemodialysis may be required. The only possible preventive measure is limiting time of manipulation of the diagnostic catheters and guidewires in the aorta. When manifestations of this complication are diffuse, involving different arterial fields, mortality is very high.

Infection

Microbial infections, local or systemic, are rare if the appropriate antiseptic technique is applied pre-, during, and postprocedure. Antimicrobial drug prophylaxis is not recommended for cardiac catheterization. It may be considered for immunocompromised patients and for any patient with probable or definite wound contamination during the procedure. The operator should avoid accessing a site where skin is not intact. It is also of utmost importance for a patient to follow postcardiac catheterization recommendations and restrictions outlined for him/her in order to minimize the risk of infection. If infection still occurs, it usually manifests itself with local pain at the access site, erythema and swelling, presence of purulent discharge from the site, fever, and elevated white blood count with left shift on differential blood count. In immunocompromised patients, some of the aforementioned clinical signs of infection may be absent. If the patient is diagnosed with systemic or local infection as a result of the procedure, empiric antibiotic therapy should be started to cover *Staphylococcus epidermidis* and *S. aureus*. Antibiotic therapy for gram-negative organisms may be added, especially if the patient is immunocompromised, has neutropenia or has other risk factors for gram-negative organisms. Compared to manual compression, infections associated with vascular closure devices tend to manifest later, be more severe with abscess formation requiring surgical drainage, device removal and arterial reconstruction in addition to systemic antibiotics.

Radiation Dermatitis

This complication occurs rarely with diagnostic cardiac catheterization, and mostly is seen in long, complex cases, including patients with multiple coronary bypass grafts. Patient notification, chart documentation, and communication with the primary care provider should routinely occur following procedures with radiation dose levels exceeding total air kerma at the reference point of ≥ 5 Gray. The cumulative dose required to cause chronic skin changes is ≥ 10 Gray (1 Gray = 100 radon). Erythema of the skin, which usually develops after it has been exposed to ≥ 10 Gray, may take several days until occurrence. Necrosis of the skin is seen with exposure of > 15 Gray. With long-term exposure to x-ray radiation chronic skin changes and cataracts may develop.

Postprocedure patient follow-up is suggested based upon assessment of dose as follows: If total air kerma > 5 Gray, patients should be educated regarding potential skin changes (e.g., a red patch on the back). Patients should be contacted at 30 days. If total air kerma > 5 but < 10 Gray, an office visit should be arranged if an adverse skin effect is suspected for better assessment by history and physical examination. If suspected, the patient should be referred to a specialist and made aware of potential radiation etiology. If total kerma ≥ 10 Gray but < 15 Gray, the patient should return for an office visit at 2 to 4 weeks with examination for possible skin effects. Finally, if total kerma ≥ 15 Gray, hospital risk management should be contacted within 24 hours with appropriate notification to the regulatory agencies.

Renal Complications

Contrast nephropathy is usually defined as a 25% increase in serum creatinine above the baseline value, or an absolute increase > 0.5 mg/dL at 48 hours after exposure to iodine contrast dye.[14] Peak elevation of serum creatinine is usually seen within 72 to 96 hours post procedure, and may take up to 7 days to return to baseline. The mechanism of acute renal injury associated with contrast dye injection is still not completely understood but seems to be multifactorial. The risk of developing this complication varies dramatically between low-risk and high-risk patients. There are several ways to assess baseline risk for developing contrast nephropathy based on clinical risk predictors (Tables 17.9 and 17.10).

When the risk score is > 4 points on precatheterization evaluation, the use of prophylactic measures (Table 17.11) is highly recommended.

TABLE 17.9   Calculating the risk score.

RISK FACTOR	POINT SCORE
Creatinine clearance < 60 mL/min	2
Use of IABP	2
Urgent or emergent procedure	2
Diabetes mellitus	1
Heart failure	1
Peripheral vascular disease	1
Use of > 260 mL contrast	1

The cumulative total of all factors' points indicates level of risk on a scale of 0 (low risk of renal complications) to 10 (highest risk of renal complications).

TABLE 17.10   Validating the risk score.

RISK SCORE	NEPHROPATHY RATE
0–4	0.2%
5–6	2.6%
7–8	8.2%
9–10	25.4%

TABLE 17.11 Prophylactic measures used to decrease the risk of CIN.

- Minimize use of contrast dye
- Use nonionic, iso-osmolar contrast dye
- Hydrate 12 hours pre- and 12 hours postprocedure with 0.45% or 0.9% normal saline
- Hold nonsteroidal anti-inflammatory drugs, and, if possible, diuretics and ACE inhibitors as well
- Optimize the hemodynamic status of patients with HF
- Delay procedure until kidney function normalizes after recent intravascular contrast dye exposure
- Consider checking serum creatinine in 48 to 72 hours postprocedure

Management of contrast nephropathy is mostly conservative with a renal consultant on board and early use of renal replacement therapy as needed.

Another important point related to contrast-induced nephropathy is the issue of lactic acidosis in patients who take metformin. Metformin is a renally excreted drug that accumulates in patients exposed to intravenous contrast dye, leading to increased production of lactic acid by the intestinal wall and reduced liver uptake. The medication should be held for 48 hours after the procedure and resumed when normal renal function is ascertained. Metformin does not need to be withheld before cardiac catheterization because, even in cases where renal dysfunction develops, the metformin level will not increase unless additional doses are taken.

References

1. Sanborn TA, Tcheng JE, Anderson HV, et al. ACC/AHA/SCAI 2014 health policy statement on structured reporting for the cardiac catheterization laboratory: a report of the American College of Cardiology Clinical Quality Committee. *Circulation*. 2014;129(24):2578-2609.

2. Byrne RA, Cassese S, Linhardt M, Kastrati A. Vascular access and closure in coronary angiography and percutaneous intervention. *Nat Rev Cardiol*. 2013;10(1):27-40.

3. Dauerman HL, Applegate RJ, Cohen DJ. Vascular closure devices: the second decade. *J Am Coll Cardiol*. 2007;50(17):1617-1626.

4. Biancari F, D'Andrea V, Di Marco C, Savino G, Tiozzo V, Catania A. Meta-analysis of randomized trials on the efficacy of vascular closure devices after diagnostic angiography and angioplasty. *Am Heart J*. 2010;159(4):518-531.

5. Patel MR, Jneid H, Derdeyn CP, et al. Arteriotomy closure devices for cardiovascular procedures. A scientific statement from the American Heart Association. *Circulation*. 2010;122:1882-1893.

6. Mego D, Thomas M, Stewart J, et al. A poly-N-acetyl glucosamine hemostatic dressing for femoral artery access site hemostasis after percutaneous coronary intervention: a pilot study. *J Invasive Cardiol.* 2010;22(1):35-39.

7. Kunert M, Gremmler B, Schleiting H, Ulbricht LJ. Use of FemoStop system for arterial puncture site closure after coronary angioplasty. *J Invasive Cardiol.* 2004;15(5):240-242.

8. Fech JC, Welsh R, Hegadoren K, Norris CM. Caring for the radial artery post-angiogram: a pilot study on a comparison of three methods of compression. *Eur J Cardiovasc Nurs.* 2012;11(1):44-50.

9. Shammas RL, Reeves WC, Mehta PM. Deep venous thrombosis and pulmonary embolism following cardiac catheterization. *Cathet Cardiovasc Diagn.* 1993;30:223-226.

10. Al-Sekaiti R, Ali M, Sallam M. Radial artery perforation after coronary intervention: is there a role for covered coronary stent? *Cathet Cardiovasc Interv.* 2011;78(4):632-635.

11. Webber GW, Jang J, Gustavson S, Olin JW. Contemporary managment of postcatheterization pseudoaneurysms. *Circulation.* 2007;115:2666-2674.

12. Tonnessen BH. Iatrogenic injury from vascular access and endovascular procedures. *Persp Vasc Surg Endovasc Ther.* 2011;23(2):128-135.

13. Blanco VR, Morís C, Barriales V, González C. Retinal cholesterol emboli during diagnostic cardiac catheterization. *Cathet Cardiovasc Intervent.* 2000;51(3):322-325.

14. Seeliger E, Sendeski M, Rihal CS, Persson PB. Contrast-induced kidney injury: mechanisms, risk factors, and prevention. *Eur Heart J.* 2012;33(16):2007-2015.

CHAPTER 18

Approach to Complex Cases in Cardiac Catheterization

"Nothing in life is to be feared. It is only to be understood."

—Marie Curie

Left Main (LM) Coronary Artery Stenosis

A diligent precatheterization work-up can help an operator to suspect the presence of left main disease, and reduce the risk of catastrophic complications of left coronary cannulation (Figure 18.1).[1,2]

Steps to be performed in the cardiac catheterization laboratory when precatheterization work-up suggests presence of LM coronary stenosis are as follows:

- **Step 1:** Crash cart is easily accessible, defibrillation pads are placed on the patient's chest, a temporary pacemaker and IABP equipment are ready to be placed if needed. An interventional cardiologist should be notified in advance about the potentially high-risk diagnostic cardiac catheterization procedure. The operator should not plan to perform cardiac catheterization on high-risk patients at the end of the day. Nonionic contrast should be used.
- **Step 2:** When a JL coronary catheter is used to cannulate the LCA, extra caution should be exercised to avoid an unintended engagement of the LCA ostium by the catheter tip when the guidewire is removed. The operator should advance the catheter tip over the guidewire deep into the cusp or stop in the mid-ascending

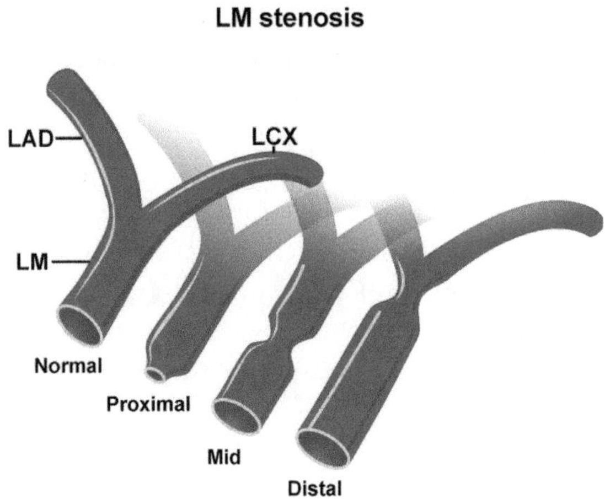

LM stenosis

FIGURE 18.1 The diagram shows various types of left main stenosis.

aorta superior to the LCA ostium. This maneuver secures careful approach to the LM coronary artery from below or above under continuous pressure monitoring. Nonselective cusp injection of contrast in shallow RAO projection with minimal caudal angulation or shallow LAO projection with minimal cranial angulation is highly recommended to visualize the ostium of the LM prior to catheter engagement.

- **Step 3:** When the catheter tip has engaged the coronary ostium, pressure waves are checked to make sure that no damping or ventricularization of the pressure waveform has occurred, as ECG tracings and the patient's clinical condition are closely monitored. If pressure damps and/or ventricularizes upon engagement of the LM, ostial stenosis is very likely. The operator should withdraw the catheter slightly, recheck the pressure waveform, then inject about 2 mL contrast gently while taking cine images. If the problem is ostial LM stenosis, an attempt can be made to gently reposition the catheter tip to eliminate pressure damping. Performing nonselective angiography or using a "hit and run" technique, where 4–6 mL of contrast dye is injected in RAO caudal and LAO cranial views with biplane angiography, are highly recommended. Alternatively, rapid rotational angiography from shallow RAO caudal or shallow LAO cranial projections to RAO cranial view can be performed with simultaneous catheter withdrawal into the ascending aorta. Aortic pressure is compared with the pressure obtained from the LM ostium and the gradient recorded. These views and information are usually sufficient to provide the cardiothoracic surgeon with a roadmap for CABG surgery. Additional injections should be avoided since frequent LM cannulations can lead to vasospasm or plaque rupture/dissection with catastrophic consequences.

- **Step 4:** If the patient's condition remains stable, the operator proceeds with right coronary angiography. For the patient with significant LM stenosis with occluded and/or a small and nondominant right coronary artery, admission to the ICU is recommended. Any patient with clinical symptoms of ischemia or even with minor signs of hemodynamic instability requires immediate IABP placement and urgent cardiothoracic surgery and interventional cardiology consultations.

Coronary Anomalies

The most frequent coronary anomaly observed during selective coronary angiography is the absence of a LM coronary artery, with the LCX and LAD either sharing a common origin from the aorta but splitting immediately, or originating separately in the left coronary cusp (LCC).[2,3] When approached with a JL coronary catheter, the tip may selectively engage either the LAD or LCX. Most of the time it is difficult to opacify both arteries simultaneously, and each artery should be cannulated separately. Occasionally, it can be accomplished by rotating the JL catheter counterclockwise in order to engage the LAD, and clockwise to get the LCX. Sometimes the catheter needs to be changed according to a simple rule: If the LCX artery is engaged on the initial attempt with the JL4 catheter, the operator should use a JL3.5 catheter to get the LAD, and vice versa (e.g., if the smaller-curve JL catheter engages the LAD, a larger-curve catheter is used to engage the LCX). If the above approach does not yield adequate information, other catheters, including the AL or MP (technique described in Chapter 7), should be considered.

The LM coronary artery occasionally may be difficult to cannulate by a preformed JL coronary catheter, despite originating from the LCC, when the ostium is either deep down or high up in the cusp, or when it is posteriorly or anteriorly oriented. A nonselective "cusp" shot frequently helps the operator to visualize the origin of the LM and choose the appropriate catheter and approach. Usually, an anomalously originating LM coronary artery located in the left coronary sinus can be approached and successfully

A

LCA from RCC

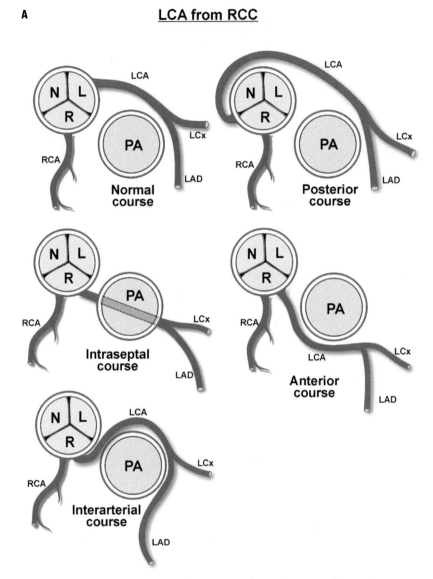

FIGURE 18.2   Coronary anomalies of the LCA (**Panel A**) and RCA (**Panel B**) are shown.

cannulated by the MP or AL coronary catheters (counterclockwise rotation for posterior location, and clockwise rotation for anterior position). A LM originating from the right sinus of Valsalva is rare (0.15% of patients), and even more rare when originating from the noncoronary sinus.[3] Figure 18.2 depicts some of the most common coronary anomalies in adults.

B **RCA from LCC**

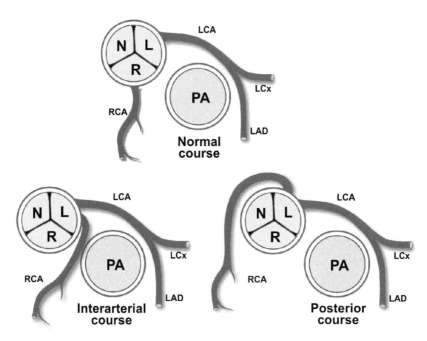

FIGURE 18.2   Coronary anomalies of the RCA (**Panel B**) (*Continued*)

WHICH ANOMALIES ARE DANGEROUS?

When the LM or RCA originates from the noncoronary sinus, its course is benign and not associated with major adverse effects. A LM originating from the right sinus of Valsalva is somewhat more problematic. The course of the artery is not necessarily benign, since it can run between the PA and aorta, a course that can be associated with sudden cardiac death. In general, cannulation of the LM originating from the right sinus of Valsalva is accomplished using AR or AL coronary catheters. The origin of the LM anteriorly to the ostium of the RCA, on the other hand, is usually a dangerous course. The same can be said about the anomalous origin of the LAD artery from the right sinus of Valsalva. On the other hand, an anomalous origin of the LCX from the right sinus of Valsalva is always followed by a benign course, although the risk of developing atherosclerosis may be higher. This type of an anomalous origin can be cannulated using modified AR or MP catheters.

Occasionally, the LCX shares a common ostium with the RCA and can be opacified with a JR catheter. When the RCA originates from the left sinus of Valsalva, its course can also frequently be malignant, especially if its ostium is anteriorly located in relation to the LM ostium. To selectively cannulate this artery, the operator may consider using JL5 or JL6, AR, or AL coronary catheters.

Referral to CT angiography in case of a suspected malignant course of an anomalous left or right coronary artery is highly recommended. The RCA origin in the right sinus of Valsalva can also vary: An inferior ectopic origin can be most successfully cannulated with a MP catheter; an anterior ectopic origin in the cusp is best cannulated with AL or AR catheters; a posterior ectopic origin can be cannulated best with an MP catheter; a superior/anterior ectopic origin above the sinotubular junction is best approached with MP (see Chapter 7), AL, or 3D-RCA coronary catheters. When using a 3D-RCA catheter, the operator should slowly withdraw the catheter into the ascending aorta from the cusp with minimal clockwise rotation and frequent test injections to orient the tip of the catheter towards the coronary ostium.

Test injections of contrast are used with attempts to cannulate any anomalous coronary vessel with clockwise or counterclockwise maneuvers of the catheter. For example, if the anomalous coronary artery is located more anteriorly, step-by-step clockwise rotation with test injections will opacify the artery gradually, since the tip of the catheter will be approaching the ostium. On the other hand, step-by-step counterclockwise rotations with nonselective test injections will poorly opacify the same artery, since the tip of the catheter will be pointing away posteriorly from the ostium. Similarly, small, nonselective test injections are helpful when the operator attempts to determine if the ostium of the anomalous coronary artery is located high or low in the cusp. In order to evaluate the course of an anomalous coronary artery arising from another (anomalous) cusp, an operator should take an RAO view. If the initial course of the coronary artery is posteriorly directed, the course is more likely to be "benign", on the other hand if the initial course of the artery is anteriorly directed the course is more likely to be "malignant".

Coronary Spasm and Myocardial Bridge

The decision to further investigate a patient with angiographically normal coronary arteries or with physiologically insignificant stenosis is made when the clinical suspicion of coronary vasospasm causing myocardial ischemia is high based on the combination of

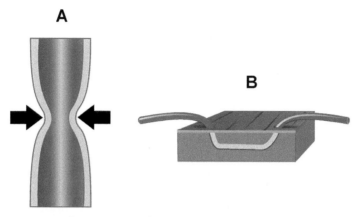

FIGURE 18.3   **Panel A** is a diagram of coronary vasospasm; **Panel B** is an example of myocardial bridging.

subjective (history and physical) and objective data (ECG and non-invasive cardiac imaging) (Figure 18.3A).[4,5] Occasionally, the simple cannulation of the coronary artery or a simple, forced episode of hyperventilation in patients predisposed to coronary vasospasm may provoke vasospasm that can be directly visualized by selective coronary angiography and resolved by intracoronary administration of nitroglycerin. In patients with symptoms related to cold exposure, a cold pressor test (immersing hands into icy cold water) can be performed in the cardiac catheterization laboratory.

If these maneuvers do not provoke coronary vasospasm, the operator may proceed with pharmacologic provocative testing. The 2 most frequently used agents for this purpose in the United States are methylergonovine and acetylcholine. In Europe and Japan, ergonovine maleate is used as well. To reverse the effect of these medications, intracoronary nitroglycerin is administered as needed. Bradycardia and hypotension, which may follow acetylcholine infusion, can be treated by intravenous administration of atropine 0.5 mg every 3–5 minutes up to a total dose of 2 mg. Major contraindications to performing pharmacological provocative testing are severe LV dysfunction, severe aortic stenosis, amenorrhea in premenopausal women (possible pregnancy), and significant LM coronary stenosis.

Different protocols for pharmacological provocative testing have been described in the literature. Ergonovine maleate can be given intravenously at doses of 50 mcg every 5 minutes until a total maximal dose of 350 mcg; a positive response or side effects necessitate termination of the test. Ergonovine can also be given by intracoronary injection of 5–10 mcg up to a total cumulative dose of 50 mcg. Methylergonovine can be given every 3 minutes in successive intravenous boluses of 1, 2, 3, and 4 mcg/kg. Again, a positive response or side effects necessitate termination of the test. Acetylcholine can be injected in incremental doses of 20, 50, and 80 mcg every 3 minutes into the RCA, and in incremental doses of 20, 50, and 100 mcg every 3 minutes into the LCA. A positive response or side effects necessitate termination of the test. Intracoronary administration of nitroglycerin reverses vasospasm of the coronary arteries provoked by ergonovine derivatives or acetylcholine.

Epicardial coronary arteries may occasionally take an intramyo-cardial course, which may lead to the entrapment of various lengths of the artery under the myocardial tissue, described as a "bridge" (Figure 18.3B).[6] The mid-LAD followed by the RCA are most commonly involved. In general, myocardial bridging is a benign phenomenon, but in rare cases it can lead to compromised blood flow and myocar-dial ischemia. The mechanism for this complication includes systolic and more importantly diastolic compression of the vessel lumen, due to an inability or delayed ability of muscle relaxation. Furthermore, vasospasm and the development of atherosclerosis in the proximal or distal segments, just prior to, or right after the "bridge" can be contributing factors. Coronary angiography can reveal the systolic narrowing or "milking effect" of the epicardial coronary artery with or without persistent diastolic reduction in vessel lumen diameter. To assess functional significance of myocardial bridging it may be required to measure fractional flow reserve after dobutamine infu-sion or evaluate its anatomy by intravascular ultrasound. Detailed description of these methods is beyond the scope of this manual.[6]

Aortic Stenosis

When dealing with a severely calcified aortic valve, fluoroscopy of the valve in different projections can outline the orifice of the ste-notic valve and may help crossing the valve with the guidewire. To cross a severely stenotic aortic valve, a soft, straight-tipped, 0.035-inch guidewire can be used. The optimal view for crossing the aortic valve is RAO; techniques for different catheters have been described in Chapter 9. An intravenous heparin bolus (40 units/kg) should be administered after the arterial access is obtained to keep the ACT ≥ 200 seconds, with frequent (2–3 minutes) removal and cleaning of the guidewire during the procedure. The operator should never apply excessive force in an attempt to push the wire or catheter across the stenotic valve; rather, a patient trial-and-error approach with slight maneuvering of the catheter and guidewire is the way to success. Steps are as follows:

- **Step 1:** Place a 7- or 8-Fr sheath into a central vein and a 6- or 7-Fr long (90 cm) sheath (to minimize the effects of peripheral amplification, avoid manipulating iliac/abdominal aortic atherosclerosis, and allow evaluation of concomitant subaortic fixed and/or dynamic obstruction, if suspected) through the common femoral artery into the ascending aorta.
- **Step 2:** Place a Swan-Ganz catheter into the IVC. Check O_2 saturation, and advance the Swan-Ganz catheter into the SVC. Recheck O_2 saturation, and pull back into the RA, advancing the catheter into the RV and the PA while recording pressure. Then check O_2 saturation in the PA and aorta, advance the Swan-Ganz catheter into the PAWP position and record pressure, deflate the balloon, and withdraw the catheter back into the PA.
- **Step 3:** If a left-to-right shunt is suspected, do the full shunt run; otherwise, deflate the balloon, remove the Swan-Ganz catheter, and flush both sheaths.
- **Step 4:** Place a 4- to 5-Fr end-hole long (125 cm) MP catheter through the arterial sheath over the regular guidewire into the ascending aorta beyond the tip of the sheath, record arterial pressures from the tip of the MP catheter and from the femoral sheath simultaneously, and note the difference.
- **Step 5:** Use a soft-tipped, straight, long wire to cross a stenotic valve; if needed, use AL1 or AL2 catheters, and if so, use exchange J-tip guidewire to eventually exchange AL catheter to an end-hole MP. Record LV pressure followed by simultaneous pressure recording from the LV cavity and femoral sheath (50 and 100 mm/second paper speed and 0–200 mm Hg scale; 0–400 mm Hg scale can be used if needed) (Figure 18.4).

Simultaneous left ventricle and aortic pressure tracings on a "200 scale" show a mean gradient of 59 mm Hg according to the computer using the selected "shaded areas." Note that the upstroke of the LV and the aortic tracings are nearly simultaneous. This type of measurement can be obtained by doing a pull-back tracing and then superimposing the aortic and the left ventricular tracings, with the limitations of the beats not being simultaneous. When doing this, the onset of the upstrokes of each complex should be matched.

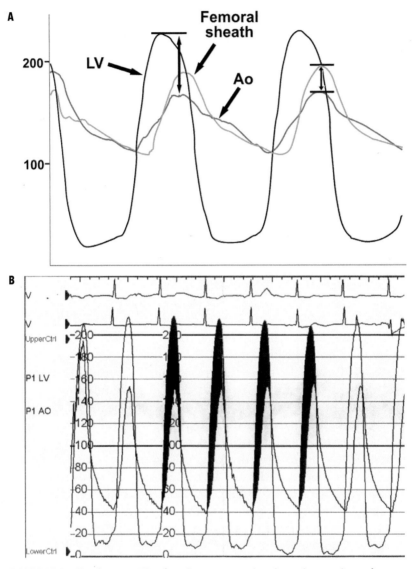

FIGURE 18.4 Simultaneous **LV** and aortic pressure tracings in aortic stenosis are shown. **Panel A**: Diagram; **Panel B**: Patient tracing.

Note the difference and add it to the delta pressure of the ascending aorta and the femoral sheath difference in order to calculate the peak-to-peak gradient, quantify the mean gradient. When done, record the peak-to-peak pressure gradient on pullback (Figure 18.5).

Left ventricle to aortic pullback tracing demonstrating a gradient of 210 mm Hg – 110 mm Hg = 100 mm Hg peak to peak.

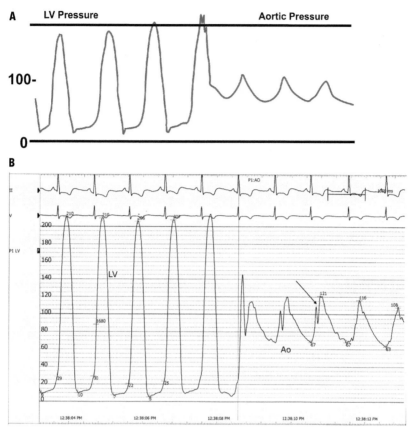

FIGURE 18.5 Pressure tracings on LV pull-back in aortic stenosis are shown. **Panel A:** Diagram; **Panel B:** Patient tracing.

Note the anacrotic notches on the aortic tracings (black arrow) and the delayed upstroke.

If the aortic pressure increases >5 mm Hg following the withdrawal of the catheter from the LV into the ascending aorta (Carabello sign),[7,8] the operator should suspect the presence of extremely severe aortic stenosis (AVA <0.7 cm²). If the operator is dealing with the clinical question of differentiation between true severe aortic stenosis versus pseudostenosis in the presence of a low transvalvular mean gradient, pharmacological (dobutamine or nitroprusside; see Box) amplification of cardiac output is used. An increase in the mean aortic gradient to ≥40 mm Hg, and an absence of significant increase of calculated aortic valve area in the presence of increased stroke volume ≥20%, suggest true aortic valve stenosis. The gradient should be measured and

PROTOCOLS FOR DOBUTAMINE AND NITROPRUSSIDE IN AORTIC STENOSIS

Dobutamine and nitroprusside protocols used in the catheterization laboratory in patients with low-output, low-gradient aortic stenosis are as follows:[7]

Dobutamine Protocol

Initiate intravenous infusion at 5.0 mcg/kg/minute and titrate every 5 minutes by 5.0 mcg/kg/min up to a maximal dose of 20 mcg/kg/minute. Measure and document the mean aortic transvalvular gradient at baseline and at the end of each stage of dobutamine infusion. Calculate and document baseline CO and SV by using the Fick equation, and repeat these calculations at the end of each stage of dobutamine infusion. The predetermined end points are: maximal dose of 20 mcg/kg/minute of dobutamine, mean gradient ≥ 40 mm Hg, increase in CO ≥ 50%, or intolerable symptoms or side effects.

Nitroprusside Protocol

Initiate intravenous infusion at 0.25 mcg/kg/minute and titrate up every 5 minutes by 0.25 mcg/kg/minute to maximal dose of 1.5 mcg/kg/minute or until mean aortic pressure is down to 65–70 mm Hg, whichever is reached first. Measure and document mean aortic transvalvular gradient at baseline and at the end of each stage of nitroprusside infusion. Calculate and document baseline CO and SV by using the Fick equation, repeat calculations at the end of each stage of the nitroprusside infusion.

averaged from 5 to 10 cardiac cycles in patients with normal sinus rhythm and atrial fibrillation respectively. If noninvasive studies have suggested concomitant subaortic fixed and/or dynamic obstruction, record simultaneous pressure tracings from the apical LV cavity and femoral sheath. Note the difference, and add to the delta pressure (femoral sheath pressure minus ascending aortic pressure) to calculate the total peak-to-peak gradient. Ask the patient to breathe out and perform the Valsalva maneuver, and record simultaneous pressures from the LV cavity and femoral sheath. When done, provoke PVCs by gently contacting the endocardium with the catheter tip, while continuing to record simultaneous pressures. If a dynamic obstruction is present, the Valsalva maneuver will lead to an increase of the existing baseline gradient; in the post-PVC beat, an increase of the pressure gradient will accompany a drop in aortic pulse pressure (Brockenbrough-Braunwald-Morrow sign) (Figure 18.6).[9]

Subsequently, record the pressure on a slow pull-back of the catheter and repeat above-described maneuvers in order to locate the site of dynamic obstruction in the LV. In case of a fixed subaortic stenosis in the LVOT, attempt to "selectively" measure the LVOT and AS gradients by moving the long sheath over the end-hole catheter into the LV and positioning it before the LVOT obstruction while the tip of the end-hole catheter is located in the

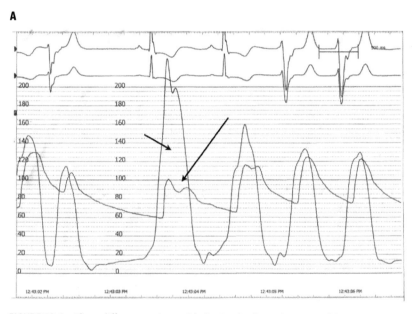

FIGURE 18.6   Three different tracings with the Brockenbrough-Braunwald-Morrow sign are shown. **Panel A**: Brokenbrough-Braunwald-Morrow sign demonstrating enhancing of the LV-to-aortic gradient **(short arrow)** and development of a "spike-and-dome" configuration to the aortic tracing **(long arrow)**. **Panel B**: Brokenbrough-Braunwald-Morrow sign with a significant LV-to-aortic gradient with a murmur demonstrated above on the phonocardiogram, followed by a premature beat and lessening of the gradient, a pause and a large gradient, a louder murmur, and the appearance of the "spike-and-dome" configuration to the aortic tracing. **Panel C**: Tracing obtained at the time of left heart catheterization with recording from the femoral sheath and the left ventricle. Sinus rhythm is present and a ventricular premature beat occurs followed by a large gradient. Short arrow indicates the aortic pressure tracing and long arrow the left ventricular tracing.

B

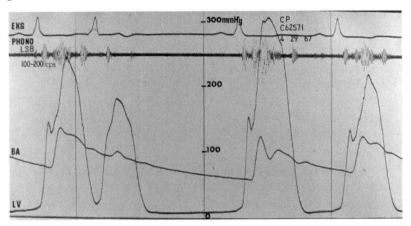

C

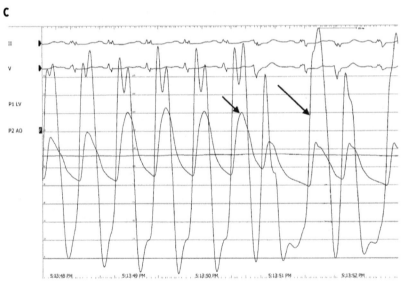

FIGURE 18.6 *(Continued)*

LV beyond the obstruction. The "selective" measurement of the AS gradient can be performed by withdrawing the sheath into the aorta while the end-hole catheter tip is positioned between the aortic valve and the LVOT obstruction.

- **Step 6:** Remove the catheter and flush both sheaths.
  - *Mild AS:* mean gradient < 25 mm Hg
  - *Moderate AS:* mean gradient 25–39 mm Hg
  - *Severe AS:* ≥ 40 mm Hg

Pulmonic Stenosis

Steps for addressing pulmonic stenosis are as follows:

- **Step 1:** Place two 7- or 8-Fr sheaths in the central vein and a 4-Fr sheath in a femoral artery.
- **Step 2:** Place a Swan-Ganz catheter into the IVC, check O_2 saturation, and advance the Swan-Ganz catheter into the SVC. Check O_2 saturation again, pull back into the RA, advance the catheter into the RV and PA (use soft-tipped, straight wire to cross the pulmonic valve), then check O_2 saturation in the PA and aorta and record PA pressure. If a shunt is suspected based on the obtained O_2 saturation values, perform a complete shunt run.
- **Step 3:** Place another Swan-Ganz catheter into the RV. Record RV pressure and then PA and RV pressures simultaneously on 50- and 100-mm/second paper speed and 0–100 mm Hg and 0–50 mm Hg scales. Measure and document the mean pressure gradient. While recording simultaneous pressures, it is critical to obtain high-quality tracings, to be able to accurately calculate the peak-to-peak and mean pressure gradients through the pulmonic valve. The gradient should be measured and averaged from 5 to 10 cardiac cycles in patients with normal sinus rhythm and atrial fibrillation, respectively. Record peak-to-peak pressure gradient on pull-back (Figure 18.7). Occasionally, an additional gradient may be detected across the infundibulum due to the presence of severe muscular hypertrophy. In such cases, the operator may consider performing right ventriculography utilizing a pigtail or Berman catheter (total 45 mL of contrast injected at 15 mL/

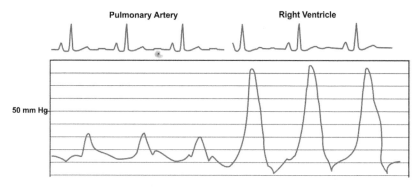

FIGURE 18.7   **Pressure tracing on pull-back in pulmonic stenosis is shown.**

second speed) in left lateral projection to visualize the infundibular obstruction.

- *Mild PS:* peak-to-peak < 30 mm Hg
- *Moderate PS:* peak-to-peak 30–60 mm Hg
- *Severe PS:* peak-to-peak > 60 mm Hg

Pulmonic regurgitation can be visualized in AP or RAO projections with 10- to 20-degree cranial angulations. Pigtail or Berman catheters are used for this purpose with total volume of the injected contrast of 50 mL at the speed of 25 mL/second.

Mitral Stenosis

When performing invasive hemodynamic evaluation of a patient with mitral stenosis in the cardiac catheterization laboratory, the operator should observe the following hemodynamic findings: increase in LA pressure, prominent "a" wave on PAWP tracing secondary to initial increment of atrial contraction, blunted "y" wave on PAWP tracing due to slowing of left ventricular filling (Figure 18.8), elevated PA pressure, and presence of a pressure gradient between mean PAWP and LVDP.[7]

On the left side of the figure, the "raw" tracings are shown, and on the right, the processed tracings. The diastolic gradient has been selected; the cardiac output is calculated using the Fick method and the computer uses the Gorlin equation to obtain a valve area

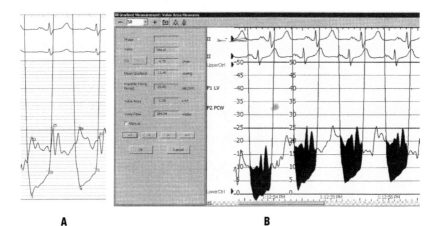

A   **B**

FIGURE 18.8   Simultaneous left ventricular and pulmonary artery wedge pressure tracings in two individuals with mitral stenosis are shown.

of 1.29 cm². Simultaneous LV/PAWP tracings are recorded on 50 mm Hg scale. Note the "p-mitrale" on the ECG tracing.

- **Step 1:** Place a 7- to 8-Fr sheath into a central vein and a 4- to 5-Fr sheath into a femoral artery.
- **Step 2:** Place a Swan-Ganz catheter into the IVC. Check O_2 saturation and advance the catheter into the SVC; check O_2 saturation and pull back into the RA; advance the catheter into the RV followed by the PA and record pressures. Then, check O_2 saturation in the PA and aorta/femoral artery and place an MP or an angled pigtail catheter into the LV cavity. Record LVEDP, advance the Swan-Ganz catheter into the PAWP position and record the PAWP, followed by simultaneous recording of the LVDP and PAWP pressures on 100-mm/second paper speed and 0–50 mm Hg pressure scale, then measure the mean pressure gradient (Figure 18.9). It is critically important to obtain high-quality

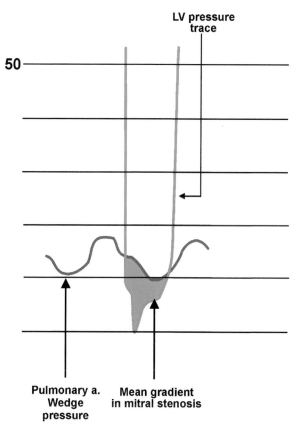

FIGURE 18.9   Tracing showing mitral stenosis (see text for details).

tracings in order to accurately calculate the mean pressure gradient while accounting for alignment mismatch between the PAWP and the LVDP. The gradient should be measured and averaged from 5 to 10 cardiac cycles in patients with normal sinus rhythm and atrial fibrillation, respectively.

- **Step 3:** If a shunt is suspected from the obtained O_2 saturation values a full shunt run should be completed.

    Ideally, the transseptal approach most accurately measures LA pressure, since the PAWP may not be an accurate representation of LA pressure with certain comorbid conditions, such as obstructive airway disease, cor triatriatum or pulmonary veno-occlusive disease.
- Normal mitral valve area (MVA): 4–6 cm²
- Mild mitral stenosis: MVA ≤ 2.0 cm²
- Moderate mitral stenosis: MVA ≤ 1.5 cm²
- Severe mitral stenosis: MVA < 1.0 cm²
- Mean MV transvalvular gradient:
    - Mild mitral stenosis: < 5 mm Hg
    - Moderate mitral stenosis: 5–10 mm Hg
    - Severe mitral stenosis: > 10 mm Hg

Tricuspid Stenosis

When performing an invasive hemodynamic evaluation of a patient with tricuspid stenosis in the cardiac catheterization laboratory, the operator expects to observe the following hemodynamic findings: increase in RA pressure, prominent "a" wave on RA pressure tracing secondary to initial increment of atrial contraction, blunted "y" wave on RA pressure tracing due to slowing of RV filling, and presence of a pressure gradient between mean RA and RV diastolic pressures.

- **Step 1:** Place two 7- or 8-Fr sheaths into the central vein and one 4-Fr sheath into the femoral artery.
- **Step 2:** Place the Swan-Ganz catheter into the IVC. Check O_2 saturation and advance the Swan-Ganz catheter into the SVC; check O_2 saturation and pull back into the RA, advance the catheter into the RV (may need to use soft tipped straight wire) and the PA. Then check O_2 saturation in the PA and aorta/femoral artery, and pull back into the RV and record RV pressure. If a shunt is suspected from the obtained O_2 saturation values, the operator needs to complete a full shunt run.

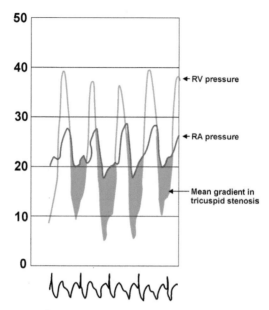

FIGURE 18.10   Tracing showing tricuspid stenosis (see text for details).

- **Step 3:** Place another Swan-Ganz catheter into the RA, record RA pressure, and then RA and RV pressures simultaneously on 100-mm/second paper speed and 0–50 mm Hg pressure scale. Measure and document the mean pressure gradient (Figure 18.10). While recording simultaneous pressures it is critical to obtain high-quality tracings in order to calculate the mean pressure gradient through the tricuspid valve. The gradient should be measured and averaged from 5 to 10 cardiac cycles in patients with normal sinus rhythm and atrial fibrillation, respectively.
- Normal TV area is 6–7 cm²
- Mean TV gradient ≥ 4 mm Hg will elevate the RA pressure:
  - Mild tricuspid stenosis: < 3 mm Hg
  - Moderate tricuspid stenosis: < 5 mm Hg
  - Severe tricuspid stenosis: ≥ 5 mm Hg
A TV area ≤ 1.0 cm² suggests severe stenosis.

Tricuspid Regurgitation

Tricuspid regurgitation can be visualized in the RAO view. Pigtail or Berman catheters are used for this purpose with total volume of the injected contrast of 45 mL at the speed of 15 mL/second.

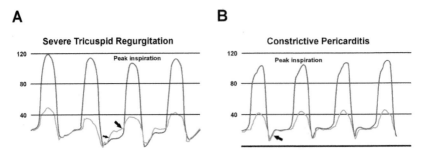

FIGURE 18.11   Hemodynamic differences between severe tricuspid regurgitation (**Panel A**) and constrictive pericarditis (**Panel B**) are shown (see text for details).

Severe tricuspid regurgitation can be differentiated from constrictive pericarditis by examining the hemodynamic tracings during deep respiration (Figure 18.11). On inspiration, the difference between the RVEDP and the LVEDP becomes more prominent with severe tricuspid regurgitation (large arrow on Figure 18.11A) and less prominent with constrictive pericarditis (arrow on Figure 18.11B). Also, the height and the slope of the RV rapid, early diastolic filling waveform become more accentuated with severe tricuspid regurgitation (small arrow on Figure 18.11A), but not in constrictive pericarditis.[10] Figure 8.12 A-C depict hemodynamic tracings of severe tricuspid regurgitation at the femoral vein, right atrium, and right ventricle.

Aortic Regurgitation

- **Step 1:** Place a long, 45-cm, 6-Fr sheath in the femoral artery.
- **Step 2:** Insert and advance a straight, pigtail catheter over the guidewire into the proximal segment of the ascending aorta, just above the sinotubular junction.
- **Step 3:** Cross the aortic valve with the pigtail catheter and record simultaneous pressures from LV and aorta (Figure 18.13). Note magnitude of LVEDP and aortic end-diastolic pressure.
- **Step 4:** Pull back pigtail catheter into the ascending aorta and place it just above the sinotubular junction. Use biplane aortography at LAO 60-degree and RAO 45-degree projections. Use 75 mL of contrast volume at injection speed of 25 mL/second with no rise. Document and grade severity of aortic regurgitation:
  - 1+ or mild AR: faint, incomplete opacification of the LV with rapid clearing

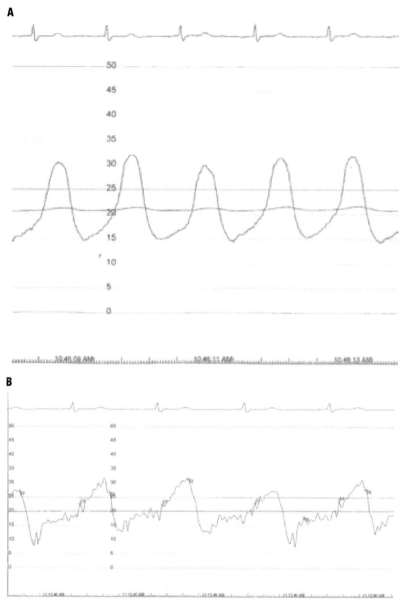

FIGURE 18.12 Hemodynamic tracings of severe tricuspid regurgitation are shown.
Panel A: Tracing obtained from transducing the sheath side port and demonstrating a large "v" wave transmitted down the inferior vena cava to the femoral vein. Pulsatile flow was noted when the femoral vein was entered with the finding needle. **Panel B**: Right atrial pressure tracing demonstrating a large, regurgitant "v" wave and a tracing very similar to the RV tracing below. This is consistent with severe tricuspid regurgitation.
Panel C: RV tracing demonstrating pressures that are close to normal and a tracing similar to the RA tracing.

C

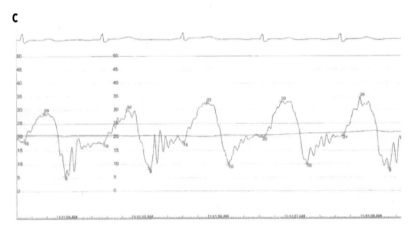

FIGURE 18.12 (*Continued*)

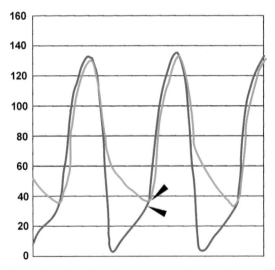

FIGURE 18.13   Hemodynamic tracing shows acute aortic regurgitation with equalization of LV and aortic end-diastolic pressures (see text for details).

- 2+ or moderate AR: faint, complete opacification of the LV with rapid clearing
- 3+ or moderate to severe AR: equal aortic and LV opacification with intermediate clearing
- 4+ or severe AR: greater LV than aortic opacification with slow clearing

Mitral Regurgitation

- **Step 1:** Place a 6-Fr sheath into the femoral artery.
- **Step 2:** Place a 7- to 8-Fr sheath into the femoral vein.
- **Step 3:** Place a Swan-Ganz catheter into the PA.
- **Step 4:** Insert and advance a 6-Fr angled pigtail catheter over the wire into the LV.
- **Step 5:** Advance the Swan-Ganz catheter into the PA wedge position.
- **Step 6:** Record simultaneously PAWP and LVEDP on 50 mm Hg pressure scale (Figure 18.14).
- **Step 7:** Use biplane mode for left ventriculography in LAO 45-degree view with cranial angulation and RAO 45-degree views. Use 50 mL of contrast at injection speed of 12–15 mL/second, with a rate rise of 0.4 and a pressure of 600 PSI.

Document and grade severity of MR:
- 1+ or mild MR: the LA clears with each beat; entire LA is never opacified
- 2+ or moderate MR: the LA does not clear with a single beat; may faintly opacify the entire LA
- 3+ or moderate to severe MR: fills the entire LA over 2 or 3 beats; equal opacification of LA and LV
- 4+ or severe MR: complete and dense opacification of the LA in one beat; contrast material refluxes into pulmonary veins

Hypertrophic Cardiomyopathy

Patients with hypertrophic cardiomyopathy can be classified into 3 major groups based on hemodynamic assessment:

1. Patients with left ventricular obstruction at rest: peak-to-peak gradient ≥ 30 mm Hg.
2. Patients with significant, dynamic left ventricular obstruction: peak-to-peak gradient ≥ 50 mm Hg with provocation.
3. Patients without significant left ventricular obstruction: peak-to-peak gradient < 30 mm Hg at rest and with provocation.

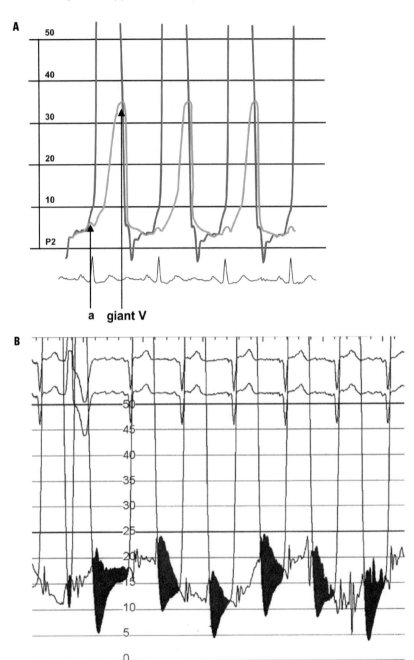

FIGURE 18.14 Hemodynamic tracing of mitral regurgitation is shown (see text for details). **Panel A**: Large "v" wave on PAWP tracing (**blue**); **Panel B**: Patient tracing. Simultaneous tracings from the left ventricle and the pulmonary capillary wedge position demonstrating a mildly elevated "v" wave indicating some degree of mitral regurgitation, but no gradient at the end of diastole, indicating the absence of mitral stenosis.

Evaluation of hypertrophic obstructive cardiomyopathy in the cardiac catheterization laboratory may be undertaken using the following steps:

- **Step 1:** Place a 6- to 7-Fr, long (45–60 cm) sheath in the common femoral artery. Obtain O_2 saturation in the SVC.
- **Step 2:** Place a 4- to 5-Fr, end-hole MP catheter through the arterial sheath into the proximal segment of the ascending aorta. Record the pressures from the tip of the MP catheter and the femoral sheath simultaneously and note the difference. Also pay attention to the presence of "spike-and-dome" configuration (rapid systolic rise followed by mild drop in pressure, followed by a secondary peak (Figure 18.15) on the pressure tracing.
- **Step 3:** Cross the aortic valve, place the end-hole MP catheter deep into the LV cavity, and record LV pressure followed by simultaneous measurement of pressure tracings from the LV and the femoral sheath. Note the baseline difference in pressure if present, and add the delta pressure (femoral sheath pressure minus ascending aortic pressure) in order to calculate the peak-to-peak gradient. Ask the patient to breathe out and perform Valsalva maneuver and record

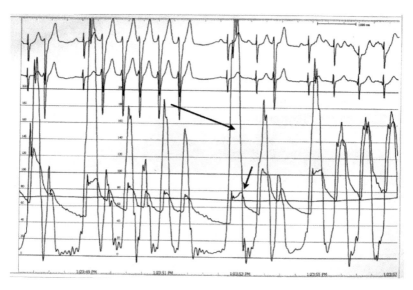

FIGURE 18.15 This recording was made during left heart catheterization with recordings from the femoral sheath and the left ventricle. Note the run of ventricular tachycardia that is probably catheter induced. After the 5-beat run, there is a pause and on the next beat or post extrasystolic beat the left ventricular pressure goes very high, off the 200 mm Hg scale (**long arrow**) and the femoral arterial pressure demonstrates a bisferiens pulse or a "spike and dome" configuration (**short arrow**).

simultaneous pressures from the LV and the femoral sheath. When done, provoke PVC by touching the endocardium with the catheter tip, while continuing to record simultaneous pressures (50- and 100-mm/second paper speed and 0–200 mm Hg pressure scale; 0–400 mm Hg scale can be used if needed). If a dynamic obstruction is present, the Valsalva maneuver will lead to the detection of the gradient or an increase of the existing baseline gradient. In the post-PVC beat, a de novo or an increase of the pressure gradient is accompanied by a drop in the aortic pulse pressure (Brockenbrough-Braunwald-Morrow sign) (Figure 18.16).[9] Record pressure on slow catheter pull-back and repeat the maneuvers described earlier to locate the site of LV obstruction. The gradient generally disappears before crossing the aortic valve unless valvular aortic stenosis is present. Occasionally, the gradient can be revealed by combining the Valsalva maneuver with PVC provocation.

- **Step 4:** If LVEDP is not > 30 mm Hg, left ventriculography can be performed to (1) reveal the presence and assess the severity of mitral regurgitation, and (2) document banana-like appearance of the LV during ventricular systole in the presence of significant LVOT obstruction. Spade-like appearance of the LV during ventricular systole is suggestive of apical hypertrophic cardiomyopathy (Yamaguchi variant).
- **Step 5:** Remove the catheter, flush the sheath, and proceed with selective coronary angiography. Occasionally, in the presence of severe septal hypertrophy, coronary angiography may show marked systolic compressions of septal coronary branches, and "sawfish" type systolic narrowing of the left anterior descending

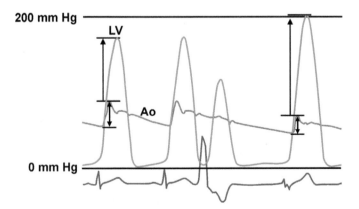

FIGURE 18.16 Hypertrophic cardiomyopathy and Brockenbrough-Braunwald-Morrow Sign are seen in this tracing (see text for details).

artery. Another finding in patients with hypertrophic cardiomyopathy may be presence of myocardial bridging.

Ideally, the transseptal approach is more accurate in recording LV pressure in order to avoid catheter entrapment and leaning of the anterolateral leaflet of the mitral valve on the catheter. Furthermore, provocative maneuvers such as amyl nitrite inhalation and isoproterenol infusion can also be utilized. Finally, when performing selective coronary angiography, optimal angiographic views of the septal arteries of the LAD are of utmost significance in order to evaluate candidacy for alcohol septal ablation as an alternative strategy to surgical septal myectomy.

Cardiac Tamponade

When the diagnosis of cardiac tamponade is established, the only effective therapy is evacuation of the content of the pericardium as quickly as possible. Ideally, this procedure should be performed in the cardiac catheterization laboratory.[11] For detailed description of the procedure, review Chapter 14.

Steps to perform in a cardiac catheterization laboratory when treating a patient with a suspected cardiac tamponade are as follows:

- **Step 1:** Cannulate the central vein (IJ, or Femoral) and place a 7- to 8-Fr sheath. Obtain O_2 saturation in the SVC.
- **Step 2:** Cannulate the femoral artery and place a 4-Fr sheath and record the pressure tracing (note pulsus paradoxus) (Figure 18.17A).
- **Step 3:** Insert a Swan-Ganz catheter into the RA and record the pressure tracing (note "y"-wave blunting and an elevated RA pressure) (Figure 18.17B).
- **Step 4:** Advance the Swan-Ganz catheter into the RV, then to the PA, and then to PA wedge position. As the catheter advances, record pressure in each chamber (note the equalization of diastolic pressures); obtain O_2 saturations in the PA and FA (to calculate CO by Fick); leave the Swan-Ganz catheter in the PA.
- **Step 5:** Place the patient at a 30- to 45-degree angle, access the pericardial space, and place a pigtail draining catheter into the pericardial space. Record simultaneously the pericardial pressure (Pp) and PAWP; Pp and PAP; Pp and RVP; Pp and RAP (slow speed, 50 mm/second and at 0–50 mm Hg pressure scale). Note

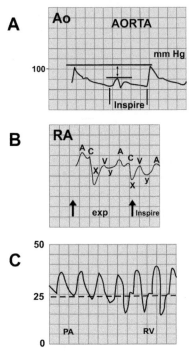

FIGURE 18.17 Hemodynamic tracings in a patient with cardiac tamponade (see text for details) are as follows: **Panel A**: pulsus paradoxus; **Panel B**: blunting of "y" wave; **Panel C**: equalization of diastolic pressures.

equalization of cardiac diastolic pressures with pericardial pressure (Figure 18.17C).

- **Step 6:** Drain the pericardial fluid completely; recheck CO by the Fick method and record right heart pressures and document the shape of the pressure tracings. If pressure tracings suggest constrictive physiology, the diagnosis of effusive–constrictive pericarditis is established.

Restrictive Cardiomyopathy versus Constrictive Pericarditis

Despite significant progress in noninvasive imaging, the differential diagnosis between constrictive pericarditis and restrictive cardiomyopathy remains difficult (Table 18.1) and frequently requires cardiac catheterization with meticulous evaluation of right and left heart hemodynamics.[7]

TABLE 18.1   Constrictive pericarditis versus restrictive cardiomyopathy.

HEMODYNAMIC SIGNS	PURE CONSTRICTION	PURE RESTRICTION
RV systolic pressure ≤ 50–55 mm Hg	(+)	(−)
LVEDP − RVEDP < 5 mm Hg	(+)	(−)
RVEDP > RV systolic pressure/3	(+)	(−)
Systolic area index* > 1.1	(+)	(−)
↓ difference between LVDP and mean PAWP with inspiration	(+)	(−)
RA mean pressure ↓ < 5 mm Hg with inspiration	(+)	(−)
LV rapid filling wave ≤ 7 mm Hg	(+)	(−)

*The systolic area index is defined as the ratio of the RV area (mm Hg × second) to the LV area (mm Hg × second) in inspiration versus expiration.

Steps to perform in the cardiac catheterization laboratory when evaluating a patient with restrictive versus constrictive cardiomyopathy are as follows:

- **Step 1:** Cannulate the central vein (IJ or Femoral) and place a 7- or 8-Fr sheath.
- **Step 2:** Cannulate the femoral artery and place a 4-Fr sheath and record arterial pressure.
- **Step 3:** Place a Swan-Ganz catheter into the RA, and record pressure (note prominent "a"-wave, prominent "x"-wave descent, sharp "y"-wave descent and elevated RA pressure) (Figure 18.18).
- **Step 4:** Advance the Swan-Ganz catheter into the RV, PA, and at the PAW position. As the catheter advances, record pressure at each site. Note the shape of the pressure tracings in the RV; look for the "square root" sign; occasionally, a negative RV early diastolic pressure can be observed in pure constrictive pericarditis. At the PAW position, record simultaneously PAWP and RAP from the distal and proximal ports of the thermodilution Swan-Ganz catheter and check for respiratory discordance. Leave the Swan-Ganz catheter in the PA and measure O_2 saturation in the PA and the femoral artery in order to calculate CO by Fick.
- **Step 5:** Advance an angled pigtail catheter over the guidewire through the femoral artery sheath into the LV cavity and record LV pressure. Then simultaneously record (slow speed, 50 mm/second and at 0–50 mm Hg pressure scale) LV and PAWP, LV and PAP, LV and RV pressures, first on 0–50 mm Hg then on 0–200 mm Hg pressure scales. Finally, measure LV and RA pressures on 0–50 mm Hg pressure scale. All simultaneous pressure

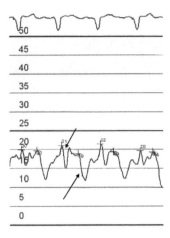

FIGURE 18.18 Right atrial pressure tracing in a patient with constrictive pericarditis shows a notable "x" descent (**short arrow**) and a prominent "y" descent (**long arrow**).

recordings should be done with unrestricted respiratory cycles (Figures 18.19 and 18.20).

- **Step 6:** Record LV–Ao gradient on pull-back; remove the pigtail catheter over the guidewire and connect the manifold directly to the arterial sheath.

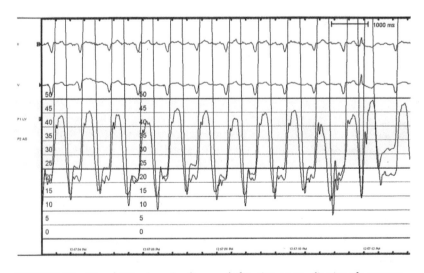

FIGURE 18.19 RV and LV tracings simultaneously focusing on equalization of pressures in diastole or at least within 5 mm Hg of each other. During inspiration, the RV pressure goes up and the LV pressure goes down.

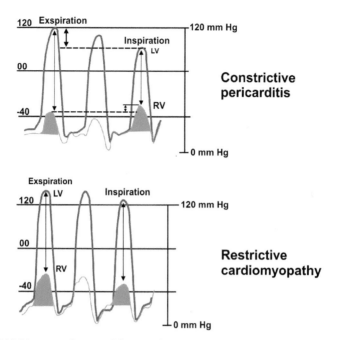

FIGURE 18.20   Hemodynamic differences between constrictive pericarditis (**Panel A**) and restrictive cardiomyopathy (**Panel B**) are shown (see text for details).

- **Step 7:** Remove the Swan-Ganz catheter, flush it, and set it aside in case repeat pressure measurements are needed.

Pulmonary Hypertension

Steps to perform in the cardiac catheterization laboratory when evaluating a patient with pulmonary hypertension are as follows:

- **Step 1:** Place a 7- or 8-Fr sheath into a femoral vein.
- **Step 2:** Place PA catheter into the PA; record and document the PAP and PAWP (measurements performed at end expiration).
- **Step 3:** If mean PAP ≥ 30 mm Hg and PVR > 3 Wood Units, place a 4-Fr sheath in the femoral artery followed by an angled pigtail catheter placement in the LV and measure LVEDP (measurement performed at end expiration). Calculate the transpulmonary gradient and CO/CI by Fick equation utilizing O_2 saturation of the Ao and PA at baseline. If the transpulmonary gradient is ≥ 15 mm Hg and the LVEDP ≤ 15 mm Hg, perform an adenosine or prostacyclin

challenge (see "Adenosine Challenge" and "Prostacyclin Challenge" Boxes). If criteria of vasoreactive pulmonary HTN is met (mean PAP drop > 10 mm Hg, and mean PAP drop to < 40 mm Hg), measure again CO/CI by Fick and document. In patients with Type 2 pulmonary hypertension nitroprusside challenge should be performed (see "Nitroprusside Challenge" Box).

ADENOSINE CHALLENGE PROTOCOL FOR ASSESSING PULMONARY VASOREACTIVITY IN PULMONARY ARTERIAL HYPERTENSION IN PATIENTS WITH MEAN PAP ≥30 MM HG AND LVEDP ≤15 MM HG

Preparation

Adenosine: Mix 4 vials of adenosine 90 mg/30 mL (total 360 mg/120 mL) into an emptied 100 mL bag of normal saline.

Infusion

Dose range: 50–400 mcg/kg/minute
Starting infusion dose: 50 mcg/kg/minute
Titration: increase dose by 50 mcg/kg/minute every 2 minutes
Maximum infusion dose: 400 mcg/kg/minute

Monitoring

BP, HR, O_2 saturation, mean PAP, cardiac output (CO) every 2 minutes. Discontinue infusion for any of the following reasons:

- SBP < 85 mm Hg or decrease in SBP > 30% from baseline
- Increase in HR > 100 bpm or > 40% from baseline
- Intolerable side effects (dizziness, dyspnea, headache, nausea)
- Bradycardia < 50 bpm associated with symptomatic hypotension
- Maximum dose of adenosine given or hemodynamic goals achieved

Hemodynamic Goals

Decrease in mean PAP by > 10 mm Hg with a mean PAP to < 40 mm Hg accompanied by normal or increased CO suggests preserved pulmonary vasoreactivity.[2] If any endpoints are reached, stop adenosine infusion while continuing monitoring.

PROSTACYCLIN CHALLENGE PROTOCOL FOR ASSESSING PULMONARY VASOREACTIVITY IN PULMONARY ARTERIAL HYPERTENSION IN PATIENTS WITH MEAN PAP ≥30 MM HG AND LVEDP ≤15 MM HG

Infusion

Dose range: 2.0–10.0 ng/kg/minute
Starting infusion dose: 2.0 ng/kg/minute
Titration: increase dose by 1.0 ng/kg/minute every 10 minutes
Maximum infusion dose: 10.0 ng/kg/minute

Monitoring

BP, HR, O_2 saturation, mean PAP continuous, cardiac output (CO) every 10 minutes. Discontinue infusion for any of the following reasons:

- SBP < 85 mm Hg or decrease in SBP > 30% from baseline
- Increase in HR > 100 bpm or > 40% from baseline
- Intolerable side effects (dizziness, dyspnea, headache, nausea)
- Desaturation and gas-exchange disturbances
- Maximum dose of prostacyclin given
- Hemodynamic goals (same as above) achieved

NITROPRUSSIDE CHALLENGE PROTOCOL FOR ASSESSING PULMONARY VASOREACTIVITY IN PATIENTS WITH TYPE 2 PULMONARY HYPERTENSION WITH MEAN PAP ≥30 MM HG AND LVEDP ≥15 MM HG

Initiate intravenous infusion at 0.25 mcg/kg/minute and titrate up every 5 minutes by 0.25 mcg/kg/minute to maximal dose of 1.5 mcg/kg/minute or until mean aortic pressure is down to 65–70 mm Hg , whichever is reached first. Measure and document LVEDP, mean aortic and pulmonary pressure at baseline and at the end of each stage of the nitroprusside infusion. Calculate and document baseline CO and SV by using the Fick equation; repeat calculations at the end of each stage of the nitroprusside infusion.

Hemodynamic Goals

Same as above.

No contraindication to adenosine or prostacyclin infusion should be present. If adenosine and prostacyclin are contraindicated, use inhaled NO (80 ppm over 10 minutes). The clinician must keep in mind that these agents could lead to an acute increase of right-to-left blood flow and potentially overload a poorly compliant LV and cause pulmonary edema. This test is contraindicated in patients with mitral stenosis or cor triatriatum.[2] No sedation is given prior to the procedure.

Simple Cardiac Shunts

Steps to perform in the cardiac catheterization laboratory when evaluating a patient with simple cardiac shunts are as follows:

- **Step 1:** Place a 7- to 8-Fr sheath in a central vein, and a 4-Fr sheath in the femoral artery.
- **Step 2:** Place a Swan-Ganz catheter in the IVC, check O_2 saturation and advance the catheter into the SVC, check O_2 saturation. Then advance to the RA and check O_2 saturation. Next, advance the catheter into the RV and check O_2 saturation. Check O_2 saturation in the main PA, in the left and right PA, and at the PAW wedge position. On the left side, check O_2 saturation in the LV and in the ascending and descending thoracic aorta.
- **Step 3:** If a shunt is suspected repeat measurements, document and analyze the obtained data.
  - ○ Level of a shunt is atrial: initial O_2 saturation step up ≥7% from SVC to RA
  - ○ Level of a shunt is ventricular: initial O_2 saturation step up ≥5% from RA to RV
  - ○ Level of a shunt is at the PA: initial O_2 saturation step up ≥5% from RV to PA
  - ○ Any Level (SVC to PA): O_2 saturation step up ≥7%
  - ○ Level of a shunt is SVC or IVC: Partial anomalous pulmonary venous return
  - ○ Level of a shunt is atrial: ASD; VSD with TR; partial anomalous pulmonary venous drainage; ruptured sinus of Valsalva; coronary fistula to RA; Gerbode defect
  - ○ Level of a shunt is ventricular: VSD; PDA with PR; primum ASD; coronary fistula to RV

- Level of a shunt is a PA: PDA (right PA O$_2$ saturation usually lower than left PA O$_2$ saturation); aorta-PA window; aberrant coronary origin from PA
- Level of a shunt is a PA: PDA (right PA O$_2$ saturation usually lower than left PA O$_2$ saturation); aorta-PA; aberrant coronary origin from PA

SHUNT ANGIOGRAPHY

- For VSD: Steep 70-degree LAO projection with 20-degree cranial angulation for mid segment of the septum or straight lateral view and RAO for anterior segment of the septum when performing ventriculography.
- For PDA: straight lateral view when performing aortography.
- For ASD: 30- to 40-degree LAO projection with 40-degree cranial angulation.
- For Gerbode defect (LV-RA shunt): 20-degree LAO projection with 40-degree cranial angulation when performing ventriculography.

References

1. El-Menyar AA, Al Suwaidi J, Holmes DR, Jr. Left main coronary artery stenosis: state-of-the-art. *Curr Probl Cardiol.* 2007;32(3):103-193.
2. Casserly IP, Messenger JC. Technique and catheters. *Cardiol Clin.* 2009;27:417-432.
3. Angelini P. Coronary artery anomalies: an entity in search of an identity. *Circulation.* 2007;115(10):1296-1305.
4. Zaya M, Mehta PK, Merz CN. Provocative testing for coronary reactivity and spasm. *J Am Coll Cardiol.* 2014;63(2):103-109.
5. Ong P, Athanasiadis A, Sechtem U. Patterns of coronary vasomotor responses to intracoronary acetylcholine provocation. *Heart.* 2013;99:1288-1295.
6. Corban MT, Hung OY, Eshtehardi P, et al. Myocardial bridging: contemporary understanding of pathophysiology with implications for diagnostic and therapeutic strategies. *J Am Coll Cardiol.* 2014;63(22):2346-2355.
7. Nishimura RA, Carabello BA. Hemodynamics in the cardiac catheterization laboratory of the 21st century. *Circulation.* 2012;125(17):2138-2150.
8. Carabello BA, Barry WH, Grossman W. Changes in arterial pressure during left heart pullback in patients with aortic stenosis: a sign of severe aortic stenosis. *Am J Cardiol.* 1979;44(3):424-427.
9. Brockenbrough EC, Braunwald E, Morrow AG. A hemodynamic technique or the detection of hypertropic subaortic stenosis. *Circulation.* 1961;23:189-194.

10. Jaber WA, Sorajja P, Borlaug BA, Nishimura RA. Differentiation of tricuspid regurgitation from constrictive pericarditis: novel criteria for diagnosis in the cardiac catheterisation laboratory. *Heart.* 2009;95(17):1449-1454.

11. Meltser H, Kalaria VG. Cardiac tamponade. *Catheter Cardiovasc Interv.* 2005;64(2):245-255.

CHAPTER 19

Useful Formulae and Normal Values

"But in my opinion, all things in nature occur mathematically."

—René Descartes

MEAN ARTERIAL PRESSURE (MAP) AND PULSE PRESSURE

$MAP = 1/3 \times SBP + 2/3 \times DBP$
Pulse pressure $= SBP - DBP$

CARDIAC SITE	NORMAL PRESSURE RANGE
LVEDP	4–12 mm Hg
PAWP mean	2–12 mm Hg
PAP "a" wave	3–15 mm Hg
PAP "v" wave	2–12 mm Hg
PAP mean	10–16 mm Hg
PAP systolic	16–30 mm Hg
PAP diastolic	4–12 mm Hg
RVSP	16–30 mm Hg
RVEDP	1–8 mm Hg
RAP mean	1–7 mm Hg
RAP "a" wave	2–8 mm Hg
RA "v" wave	2–8 mm Hg

CARDIAC OUTPUT (CO), CARDIAC INDEX (CI), STROKE VOLUME (SV), STROKE VOLUME INDEX (SVI), AND EJECTION FRACTION (EF)

SV = LVEDV − LVESV	Normal SV = 70–95 mL Normal LVESVI = 20–35 mL/m²
SVI = SV/BSA	Normal SVI = 35–60 mL/m²
CO = SV × HR	Normal CO = 5.2–7.5 L/minute
CI = CO/BSA	Normal CI = 2.6–4.2 L/minute/m²
EF = LVEDV − LVESV/LVEDV	Normal EF = 60–75% Normal LVEDVI = 60–90 mL/m²

SYSTEMIC (SVR) AND PULMONARY VASCULAR RESISTANCE (PVR)

SVR = (MAP − CVP)/CO	Normal SVR = 800–1,600 dynes/second/cm^{-5} 10–20 Wood Units
PVR = (mean PAP − PAWP)/CO	Normal PVR = 40–130 dynes/second/cm^{-5}, or 0.5–1.6 Wood Units

SIMPLIFIED FORMULA FOR INTRACARDIAC LEFT-TO-RIGHT SHUNT CALCULATION

Qp/Qs = (arterial O_2 saturation − mixed venous O_2 saturation)/(PAWP O_2 saturation − PA O_2 saturation)
Qp − Qs = volume of simple left-to-right shunt
Qs − Qp = volume of simple right-to-left shunt

CARDIAC OUTPUT (CO) CALCULATION

CO systemic = O_2 consumption/13.4 × Hgb × (arterial O_2 saturation − mixed venous O_2 saturation)
CO pulmonary = O_2 consumption/13.4 × Hgb × (PAWP O_2 saturation − PA O_2 saturation)
Mixed venous O_2 sat = (3 × SVC O_2 saturation + IVC O_2 saturation)/4
O_2 consumption = Body weight (kg) × 3; O_2 consumption range = 110–150 mL/minute/m²
O_2 consumption = Body surface area (kg) × 126

CARDIAC SITE	O_2 SATURATION NORMAL RANGE
Aorta	92%–98%
LV	92%–98%
LA	92%–98%
PAWP	92%–98%
PA	65%–85%
RV	65%–85%
RA	65%–85%
SVC	65%–75%
IVC	65%–87%

If O_2 saturation step-up is > 7% from SVC to PA, suspect left-to-right shunt

Valve Area:
Gorlin Formula for:

Aortic valve area (cm²) = CO mL/minute / (44.5 × systolic flow time sec × HR beats per min × $\sqrt{\text{mean aortic valve pressure gradient}}$)

Mitral valve area (cm²) = CO mL/minute / (37.5 × diastolic flow time sec × HR beats per min × $\sqrt{\text{mean mitral valve pressure gradient}}$)

Hakki Formula for:

Aortic valve area (cm²) = CO L/minute /$\sqrt{\text{peak-to-peak aortic valve pressure gradient}}$
- If heart rate is > 90 bpm, divide above result by 1.35.

Mitral valve area (cm²) = CO L/minute /$\sqrt{\text{mean mitral valve pressure gradient}}$
- If heart rate is < 75 bpm, divide above result by 1.35.

If significant aortic or mitral regurgitation coexists with aortic or mitral stenosis, respectively, valve area can be underestimated, so it is not recommended to use Hakki or Gorlin formulas in such cases due to underestimation of flow.

AORTIC VALVE AREA	STENOSIS SEVERITY
AVA (cm²) < 1.0 cm²	Severe aortic stenosis
AVA (cm²) ≤ 1.5 cm²	Moderate aortic stenosis
AVA (cm²) ≤ 2.0 cm²	Mild aortic stenosis
AVA (cm²) = 3.0–4.0 cm²	Normal

MITRAL VALVE AREA	STENOSIS SEVERITY
MVA (cm²) < 1.0 cm²	Severe mitral stenosis
MVA (cm²) ≤ 1.5 cm²	Moderate mitral stenosis
MVA (cm²) ≤ 2.0 cm²	Mild mitral stenosis
MVA (cm²) = 4.0–6.0 cm²	Normal

APPROXIMATE TOTAL BODY OXYGEN CONSUMPTION (ML/MINUTE) AS DETERMINED BY AGE, GENDER, AND HEART RATE					
HEART RATE (BEATS/ MIN) FEMALES AGE	51–60	61–70	71–80	81–90	91–100
36–45	120	125	140	130	
46–55	125	115	118	125	130
56–65	105	107	110	125	135
66–75	100	105	125	120	110

HEART RATE (BEATS/ MIN) MALES AGE	51–60	61–70	71–80	81–90	81–100
36–45	120	135	140	150	135
46–55	120	120	130	135	135
56–65	120	120	125	125	125
66–75	115	115	125	125	

Index

left brachial artery approach,
192–194
problems, 194–198
suboptimal timing, 194–196
IVC. *See* inferior vena cava

J
Judkins Left catheter for femoral,
brachial and radial
approaches, 57–63
Judkins Right catheter
entering the left ventricle using,
134–135
for femoral, brachial and radial
approaches, 65–68
jugular vein approach,
endomyocardial biopsy and,
170–173
jugular vein vascular access, 40–42

K
kinking, knotting, and clotting,
84–87, 113, 155

L
laboratory equipment, 5–6
LAO. *See* left anterior oblique
LCA. *See* left coronary artery
left anterior oblique (LAO)
aortography and, 139–140
coronary bypass grafts and, 109,
112, 115, 117–119
left ventriculography and,
94–96
pulmonary artery angiography
and, 142
right coronary artery
cannulation and, 96–104
left brachial artery approach,
192–194
left coronary artery (LCA)
cannulation
Amplatz Left catheter for
femoral, left brachial and
radial approaches, 63–65

angiographic views, 72, 73, 74
Judkins Left catheter for
femoral, brachial and radial
approaches, 57–63
multipurpose catheter and,
104–109
left internal mammary artery
(LIMA), 111, 120, 122–124
left main (LM) coronary artery
stenosis, 231–233
left ventricle (LV)
entering the, 130–136
indications for catheterization,
127, 129
small and horizontally
positioned, 144
left ventriculography
contraindications to, 130
multipurpose catheter and,
92, 94–96
radiologic anatomy of, 127–130
LIMA. *See* left internal mammary
artery
limb ischemia, 196–197, 225–226
LM. *See* left main
LV. *See* left ventricle

M
manifold, 19, 21, 22
manual compression, 207–209
mesenteric arteries
angiography for, 72, 75, 77–78
dissections, 81–82
metformin, 229
Micropuncture Kit, 11, 12, 13
midazolam, 26
mitral regurgitation, 253
severity, 132–133
mitral stenosis, 246–248
multipurpose catheters
basics of, 90–91, 93, 94
challenging conditions, 113
coronary bypass grafts and,
109–112
development of, 89–90